DIANA SHEA

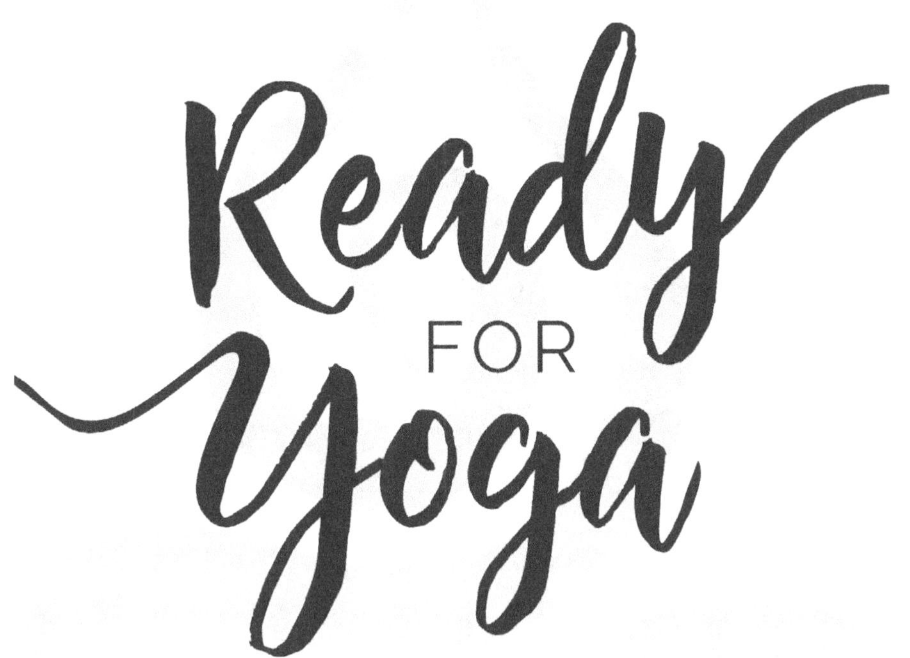

GETTING STARTED IN A WAY THAT WORKS FOR YOU

Published by CroShea Ventures, LLC

Cover design: Ida Fia Sveningsson

Interior design: Danijela Mijailovic

Tradepaper ISBN: 9781983392306

First Edition, September 2018

GET YOUR FREE *READY FOR YOGA* VIDEO HERE!

Just to say thanks for downloading my book, I would like to give you this video of me answering the five most frequently asked questions that I get about beginning a yoga practice. Packed with content, this video will jumpstart your yoga journey. Enjoy!

http://www.dianashea.com/5FAQs

Table of Contents

INTRODUCTION

Many of us want to practice yoga, but haven't yet. Why is that?

We know that yoga will reduce the amount of stress we carry around and that it will increase our flexibility. Our friends, and in some cases, our doctors, have suggested that we begin a yoga practice. We know that yoga can decrease our stress as well as our physical and mental pain and suffering. Yet we hear a voice that tells us we don't have time in our busy schedule for yoga, that we aren't flexible enough for yoga, or that we do not have the right body for yoga.

Is there a way for us to move through that resistance and quiet that voice? I believe that yoga is for every *body* and that we all have tools within us to transform our fears by rolling out a mat and giving it a try. Yoga is a healing practice and it is meant to be accessible.

These beliefs come from ten years of experience teaching yoga in a variety of environments and working with various populations, as well as three years as the director of The Yoga Centre, a private studio just outside Chicago. In that time, I have discovered that many people would like to be practicing and just need a little encouragement and gentle guidance before beginning their yoga journey. My intention with this book is to open up the world of yoga by providing a down-to-earth guide that will give more people the confidence to try it.

In this book, I am going to introduce the idea of yoga—why we practice, what yoga is, and what students can expect from a class. Together, we'll address your preconceived notions about yoga and adopt new beliefs that will serve you better. I'll share tools to clarify your desired outcome, to research local classes and to actually incorporate the practice into your life. I'll also highlight stories of everyday people who have found benefits from yoga. Perhaps you'll see a bit of yourself in them and be encouraged to move forward.

Above all else, I will show you that yoga is for you and that you can make a plan to begin.

I'm not going to tell you that beginning a yoga practice is easy or that the benefits necessarily appear right away. But I do know that if you are willing to read this book and make a plan to attend classes, you will find yourself thriving in a way that you never thought possible.

The best part is, I'll be there right along with you. I may have more yoga experience than you, but I am no stranger to the challenges of juggling a busy life while seeking greater balance. I have daily struggles to stay present when I'm cooking dinner and trying to handle my daughter's homework questions or to prioritize my own yoga practice when I am pulled between work, play and family responsibilities. When I'm under a lot of pressure, I can feel the weight on my chest and I notice that my breathing is shallow. Does that sound familiar? It's life! And we're all here to navigate the ups and downs. Yoga is just one practice that provides the tools to flourish from within and seek greater wellness no matter what the circumstances.

I honor you for picking up this book and reading to the end of this introduction in this moment. Cracking the first page of a book and taking a step toward a new experience is often the hardest part. Choosing to follow that spark within yourself requires courage. I acknowledge you for that.

The urge to write this book came from a place of knowing that the practice is meant to be welcoming. It is my hope that it will bring you closer to yoga in a way that will open up your heart and your world to the healing that it provides.

There is a place for you in this practice.

PART 1

CLARIFY YOUR INTENTION

The practice of yoga originated in India thousands of years ago. It is a system of techniques for purifying the body, both physically and mentally, including the use of the physical postures you see practiced in gyms and health clubs across the country. In many ways, we consider yoga to be synonymous with the physical practice, even though you will learn that it can include much more than that.

From the outside, it might look like yoga is just a bunch of stretching. What could possibly be the big deal about that? Turns out, the benefits of yoga go well beyond the realm of standard stretching. In Chapter 1, I will explain why we practice yoga and what benefits you can expect from the practice. I will lay out these benefits in a detailed and thorough way with the support of scientific research. If you are not convinced of the merit of yoga right now, then Chapter 1 will surely get you over that hump.

In Chapter 2, we will look more closely at what might be holding you back from the practice and shift our thought patterns so that we can create a positive image or vision for the outcome that we desire. These two pieces—aligning our thought patterns with the benefits we want from the practice—will become our personal motivation for getting on the mat, not only for the first time, but every time.

As we move through this book together, you will come across this recurring notetaking prompt as indicated by the shaded box with a cute pen. The purpose of these prompts is for you to use journaling as a way to sort through your own thoughts, as well as to keep notes for later reference. You can use a notebook, a journal, or a few pieces of paper. It need not be pretty. I have also created a printable template, should that be helpful to you (go to my website to download it: www.dianashea.com/readyforyoga). This collection of notes will become your personalized action plan for getting started, so you'll want to be sure to complete them.

THE YOGI NEXT DOOR

Another recurring section of the book is called "The Yogi Next Door", where I feature stories of everyday people that practice yoga. These stories are intended to be inspirational, to show you that it is possible to begin and that you will derive great benefit. I have sprinkled these stories throughout so that you can be continually reminded that the story could easily be your own.

Absorb them; allow them to infuse you with motivation.

Chapter 1
The Benefits of Yoga

According to a recent survey[1], the top four reasons Americans choose to start a yoga practice are flexibility (61%), stress relief (56%), general fitness (49%), and improvement of overall health (49%). My own experience with new students reflects these same motivating factors. Let's look more carefully at a few specific benefits of yoga as they relate to these reasons for getting started with yoga.

FLEXIBILITY

In my experience, greater flexibility is the single most popular reason students are attracted to yoga. Scientists have shown that weekly practice can improve flexibility in as little as six weeks[2]. In this chapter, we'll discuss a whole host of other benefits of yoga, many of which you might find even more valuable. However, the immediate and measurable effects of this practice are most easily seen with the changes in one's flexibility.

First: what is flexibility? At its core, **flexibility is made up of two parts: range of motion and mobility**. Range of motion is measured by the distance and direction your joints can move. Mobility is the ability of your muscles to move around the joints. One's own flexibility can be found within a continuum—we are not all built the same and **we do not all have equal potential for flexibility**.

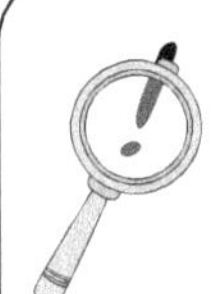

To help me explain this concept, I turned to my personal trainer, Ellen Petrick[3]. With both a master's in exercise physiology and a secondary education degree, Ellen is great at explaining things in terms we can all understand. In one of her recent classes, she talked about the flexibility continuum. Each of us is born with a certain natural range of motion and mobility, as scripted by our DNA and the unique anatomy of our connective tissue attachment points. We can all improve our flexibility by increasing the pliability of the connective tissues (through stretching), but we don't all have the capacity to reach the same levels of flexibility. As a result, **we must measure our own increase in flexibility against ourselves, not each other**. That's the first thing to know.

YOGA HACK Observe changes in your flexibility against yourself. We do not all have equal potential for flexibility, so you must not compare yourself to others. Yoga is not a competition!

The second important thing to know about flexibility is that **either end of the continuum at its extreme is undesirable**. On one end is too much flexibility or hypermobility of the joints. This can be dangerous because you have to work very hard to control your body in space and keep from hyperextending the joints (bending them in the wrong direction). On the other end of the continuum is extreme stiffness and zero range of motion due to hypertonic muscle tone, or excess muscle contraction when the muscle is not actively working.

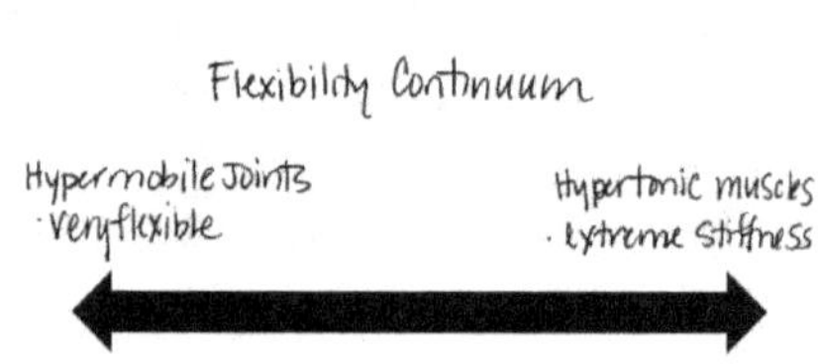

Most of us fall somewhere in between these two extremes. And thankfully, our yoga practice can inch us further up the continuum towards greater flexibility. Now, here is where a word about being good to yourself is required. We all know the difference between a stretch that is painful and a stretch that feels good. One of the main tenets of yoga is to first do no harm. With our common human orientation towards perfection, success and achievement, sometimes we forget to listen to our bodies. It is very important to acknowledge that your body has limitations and that causing yourself pain is not a good idea. You can make progress towards greater flexibility and you can do so in a safe and gentle way.

KEY POINT!

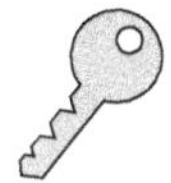

First: do no harm! Increasing flexibility
does not require pain. You can make progress
in a safe and gentle way.

Have you ever thought that you are not "good" at yoga? Well, I have news for you—**there's no such thing as being "good" at yoga!** This flexibility continuum shows that we all have different starting points. We can all work our yoga poses in a certain direction and the pose is never complete. So please don't let me hear anyone say they're not good at yoga, or that yoga is not for them. **Yoga is for every *body*.**

Along that same vein, yoga is also not a competition. You measure your own progress against yourself, no one else. Just like there's no such thing as being "good" at yoga, there's also no such thing as being "better" at yoga than someone else.

STRESS RELIEF

Yoga and meditation have long been believed, through direct experience, to aid in the reduction of stress. Today, there is an entire industry that has grown up around stress management services and education. A simple Google search will result in any number of tips and classes offering support to those who seek to lower stress. While there are many ways to reduce stress, some common suggestions include regular exercise, relaxation techniques, journaling, and talking with a friend. **Yoga is often specifically recommended to reduce stress, as it nicely blends methods of both relaxing the body and quieting the mind.**

Medical research supports this recommendation[4]. Your friends are right— yoga will reduce your symptoms of stress[5], as well as the measurable precursors to heart disease[6].

BALANCE

Balance is one of the first physical skills we start to lose quickly if we don't practice it. Going about our daily lives (not to mention maintaining an active lifestyle) requires a fair amount of balance, and we don't often appreciate it until we lose it.

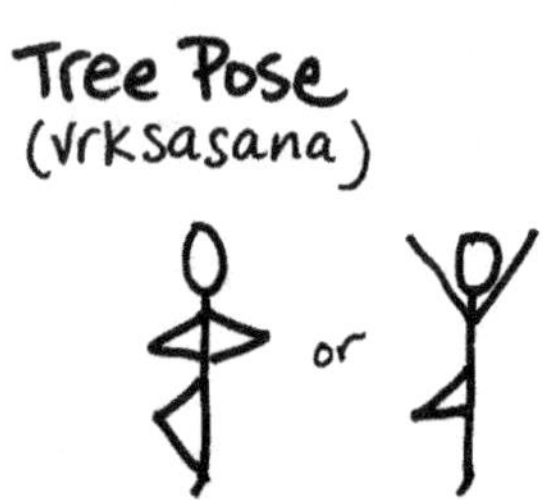

Did you know that working on the skill of balance is more than just standing on one leg (as in tree pose)? Our bodies need strength and flexibility in order to be able to handle balancing. Likewise, the full practice of yoga helps work on balance skills, instead of just those poses where your balance is challenged.

And, it's not just aging persons that can improve their balance with yoga[7]. Regular yoga practice can even improve the postural control of college athletes[8]. It's never too late or too early to work on your balance skills!

PSYCHOLOGICAL HEALTH AND WELL-BEING

One of my dear friends, Stephanie, posted this picture on Facebook of her wearing a t-shirt that says, "I'm nicer after yoga." I think she's sweet as pie all the time, but Stephanie reports definitively that she feels uplifted after a yoga class and interacts differently with those around her as a result.

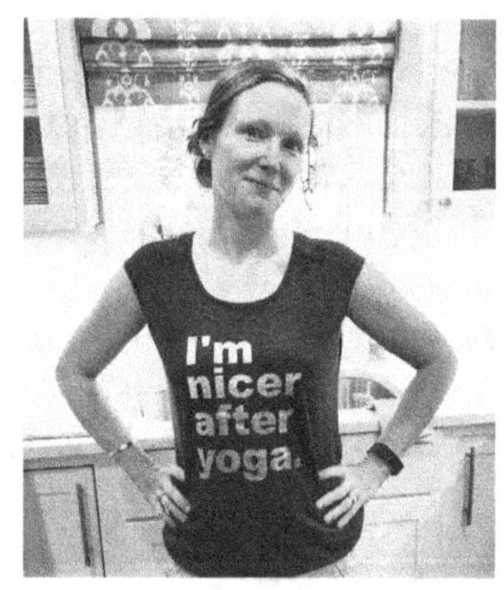

I have experienced this myself and so can you. Walking out of a yoga class. I often feel that the weight of the world is lifted off of my shoulders. I can breathe more deeply and feel more grounded.

There is science to support this too. **The practice of yoga elevates mood and improves measures of psychological health[9] [10], even more than other forms of aerobic exercise[11] [12].**

THE BOTTOM LINE

Which of these benefits gets you excited? What popped out for you as something that would really change your everyday life? You might circle the benefit that most intrigues you or follow the writing prompt below. We'll come back to this when we begin to research classes.

Which benefit of practicing yoga do you find most appealing?
Choose one or prioritize the list by numbering them from 1-4.

__FLEXIBILITY __ STRESS RELIEF __ BALANCE __ PSYCHOLOGICAL HEALTH

THE YOGI NEXT DOOR: MEET JANE

Jane started experiencing neck pain and headaches as a result of the repetitive motions and long hours that were part of her work as an ultrasonographer. When her cousin suggested that she try yoga to relieve the pain, Jane was all for it. She signed up for a one-month hatha yoga class with a certified instructor.

After the first class, Jane was less than satisfied. "I was so mad!" she says. "I thought it was boring and felt that I could be out jogging and getting more of a workout." Luckily for her, she didn't abandon yoga right away. She had paid for a full month of classes, so she was determined to stick it out.

Her persistence paid off. After one month of classes, her pain and headaches started to decline. After two months of classes, her pain and headaches had completely gone away. She was hooked.

After years of studying with a teacher, Jane now primarily practices on her own at home or with a video. She thinks that starting out with a certified instructor in a class setting was crucial for her. "I learned the correct way to do yoga from the beginning, which maximizes my results and minimizes injury." Today, Jane loves her yoga practice for maintaining flexibility and strengthening without the use of weights. Her advice to students that are new to yoga: "You have to try it to see if you like it. You might be surprised, like I was, at how wonderful it made me feel!"

Chapter 2
Empowering Beliefs

To open this next chapter, it feels important to me to first agree that life is busy and often stressful. I get it. As a mom of two young kids (and our sweet dog, Sasha!), I know how hard it is to prioritize my own health over my other responsibilities. I know how hard it can be to try new things or to feel like you don't belong. I know that the struggle is real. And yet, despite that, I'm here to tell you that you can create that which you desire. You are enough and there is enough time. Hear me out.

In this chapter, we will carefully consider why you might be experiencing resistance to practicing yoga, or what your individual challenges are with creating the time and space for it. What is the root of that resistance for you? It can come in many forms. But there's one thing that is the same no matter where your resistance comes from: in order to propel you forward into action, we need to create a stronger connection with your motivation and interest in the practice.

To do that, we will first consider your reason for being here—for taking the time to open up this book. Next, we'll take a look at what, specifically, is holding you back—those thoughts that have previously convinced you that you had no business trying yoga. We call these limiting beliefs.

Then we'll take your limiting beliefs and turn them on their head. We will transform them into empowering beliefs that will better serve you and your reason for being here. Once you've shifted your perspective, we will be able to create a vision for your practice that you can believe, through every fiber of your being. And it will drive you to figure out strategies to get there.

This is a time-tested goal-setting process that works, but it's up to you to make sure that your reason for being here is strong, because without it, you may not take the next step.

With that said, we're ready to dive in!

CONNECTING WITH PURPOSE

In my experience, the juice behind the motivation to take action is purpose. Why are you interested in learning more about yoga? What is the end result you are hoping to get out of a yoga practice? There may be more than one answer to these questions, or you might not have any answers yet. Both are OK. Let's take a minute and jot down a few of your thoughts as you answer these aforementioned prompts. **Connecting with purpose and writing it down can supercharge your desire to stick to a new practice.**

Get rooted in your desire to practice yoga by connecting with a driving force. Take a few minutes to journal your responses to the following questions:
- Why are you interested in learning more about yoga?
- What would you like to gain from developing a yoga practice?
- How would your life be different if you practiced yoga?

Not sure what I mean? Let's look at a few examples.

The Working Parent

As a working parent, you want to feel more in control of your time and energy. You are pulled in multiple directions and you desire a greater sense of calm and connectedness. In this case, perhaps we might say that you want to practice yoga **to become more mindful and bring greater awareness to your everyday activities.** The practice of yoga is a great step in this direction.

The Active Adult

In another example, let's say you want to maintain your active lifestyle, participating in recreational sports or social exercise, while avoiding injury. You might say that your primary interest in yoga is **to complement your repetitive physical activities to maintain flexibility and prevent injury.** Again, yoga would serve this purpose well, particularly if you were to identify a short daily routine for yourself.

The Involved Grandparent

Let's imagine that you have grandchildren. You want to be able to take them to the park and play on the floor with them. You want to engage with them on their level and feel confident when caring for them. In this case, we might say that your primary goal is **to remain limber enough to play with your grandchildren on the floor and stable enough to carry them**. Yoga is a very good practice for that, especially if you let the teacher know that is what you are working toward. It's also easily measurable. You'll notice a difference in your abilities very quickly.

The Person in Pain

In our last example, we will consider a person who is in chronic pain, either emotionally or physically. In this case, you want to find solutions to release the painful sensations and ease the suffering. You want to feel free from the overbearing weight of it all. The driving force for this person may be **to reduce the physical symptoms of stress and find serenity and peace.**

Do any of these examples resonate with you? Here are a few more goal statements, including the examples we just went through. Do any of them feel right for you? When you find one that works, circle it. Or take a moment to come up with your own. The personal connection with your reasons for choosing yoga is important to propel you forward.

Goal Statements

- To become more present in my everyday activities.

- To become more flexible and prevent injury.

- To remain limber enough to play with grandchildren on the floor and stable enough to carry them.

- To reduce physical symptoms of stress.

- To find serenity and peace.

- To strengthen core muscles and address back pain.

- To adopt wellness habits.

- To meet like-minded active adults.

- To elevate my mood, to have a more positive outlook.

One theme I hope you can already see is that there are many reasons to practice yoga, and all of them have merit. You might be here for all of these reasons. In my experience, choosing one in particular to identify with will make getting started easier.

KEY POINT!

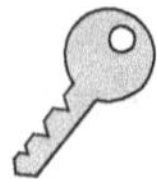

There are many very good reasons to practice yoga! Identifying one to hang your hat on can serve as a strong motivator.

Take a moment and think about what is prompting you to learn more about yoga. You are here because you have a sense that the practice will unlock some potential for you or fill an otherwise unanswered need. Once you've answered the questions above, or circled some of the sample goal statements above, you'll be ready to shift your perspective on those beliefs that are holding you back.

CREATING EMPOWERING BELIEFS

So much of our reality is created in our heads. The stories we tell ourselves are intended to help us make sense of the world around us and keep us safe. It is human nature to dislike going outside of our comfort zone. Our mind tricks us by telling stories that are designed to keep us confined within understood boundaries. I know it sounds a bit crazy. But you've probably experienced it yourself—it's just the way the mind works. These stories that we tell ourselves are comprised of our limiting beliefs.

What if we chose to use this concept to our advantage by planting the stories we wanted our brain to hear? If you have been telling yourself, "I don't have the right body for yoga", imagine how your brain chemistry changes when you tell yourself that "Yoga is for every body". You may find yourself opening up to it in a new way. You might even make it super personal. Using the same example, perhaps you turn it into, "My body is perfect for yoga." Or even further, "My beautiful body deserves the practice of yoga". Tell me that doesn't make you feel so much better!

YOGA HACK

Create an empowering belief statement about yoga to retrain your mind with a positive story about why you will practice and what you will get out of it.

There's no right answer here, except that you want to feel joy when you state your newfound belief. The point is to tap in to something in your soul that feels good and will move you forward.

In each section below, we take a closer look at those limiting beliefs that I have found to be most prominent. I have grouped them into three broad categories: not convinced of the benefit of yoga, access constraints, and feelings of intimidation. Which of these stand out to you? There may be more than one that seem to keep you off the mat entirely. Every single one of us identifies with some aspect of these, so take a look with a critical eye and ask yourself which one(s) speak to you. Select the one that seems to hold you back the most. Can you flip it around to create an empowering belief that will move you forward and confront your fears head on? I've provided some options. Feel free to use these in any form. Play with them to make them your own.

NOT CONVINCED OF THE BENEFITS OF YOGA

Limiting Belief #1: Yoga is not enough exercise for me (and maybe even a little boring). I'd rather be doing something more active, like running or spinning.

Yoga complements my other physical activities and emphasizes a mind-body connection that I don't get otherwise. I'm eager to feel the psychological benefits from yoga that have been shown to be even better than other forms of exercise.

Limiting Belief #2: Yoga is not masculine enough for me.

There are forms of yoga that are perfectly suited for me and my fitness goals. I will find classes that are geared towards men or I will build character by trying something new and being open to experiencing what it feels like to be in the minority.

Limiting Belief #3: The pseudoscience turns me off.

I will find a yoga teacher that provides instruction and commentary with proper authority based on their credentials.

FEELINGS OF INTIMIDATION

Limiting Belief #4: I don't have the right body for yoga.

Yoga is for *every body*. My beautiful body deserves the practice of yoga. I will wear whatever is comfortable for me and find a place to practice that feels good to me. There are teachers who know how to modify poses so that my body can practice with full benefit.

Limiting Belief #5: I am not good enough at yoga.

My beautiful body deserves the practice of yoga *today*, in the now. I may not be the most flexible person in the room and I'm OK with that. The teacher is there to support me, and no one is making judgments about me.

Limiting Belief #6: What if I fart in class?

Passing gas is a perfectly normal and healthy thing to do and happens sometimes (but not that often) in a yoga class. I will not judge or shame anyone for passing gas in a class I am in, and I trust that the students will respect me and my experience in the same way. I will not live my life in fear of farting!

Limiting Belief #7: The breathing part makes me nervous.

I will focus my practice on the physical postures until I feel confident enough to explore the aspects of the breath. My yoga journey does not have to begin with an awareness of the breath. I want to know more about how to follow my breath in a yoga class and I will find the perfect teacher to gently guide me.

ACCESS CONSTRAINTS

Limiting Belief #8: Yoga is expensive.

The value I place on the benefits of a yoga practice is equal to the amount I am willing to pay for it as a service. I will find a form of practice that perfectly matches my budget for it.

Limiting Belief #9: Going to yoga class takes too much time.

The value I place on the benefits of a yoga practice is equal to the amount of time I am willing to exchange for it as a service. I will find a form of practice that meets the amount of time I am willing to spend on it.

Limiting Belief #10: I don't have the support of my family.

My family wants what is best for me. I will read this book and learn more about the benefits of a yoga practice so that I can share the information with my family. We will work together to come up with strategies to get me to a class.

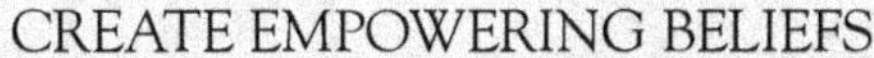

CREATE EMPOWERING BELIEFS

- What is holding you back from practicing yoga? What limiting belief stops you from trying yoga? Use an example from above or write your own.
- Flip the limiting belief on its head and rewrite it as an empowering belief. By writing it down, you will begin to create a personal connection to it.

STEPPING INTO YOUR VISION

Have I told you that you're doing a great job? I'm so proud of you for making it this far. It's not easy to critically look at our beliefs and evaluate our reasons for doing things. It's something that many of us are not in the practice of doing, so it can feel quite challenging. However, with a reason for practicing and a shift in perspective, you will be able to take the next steps more reliably.

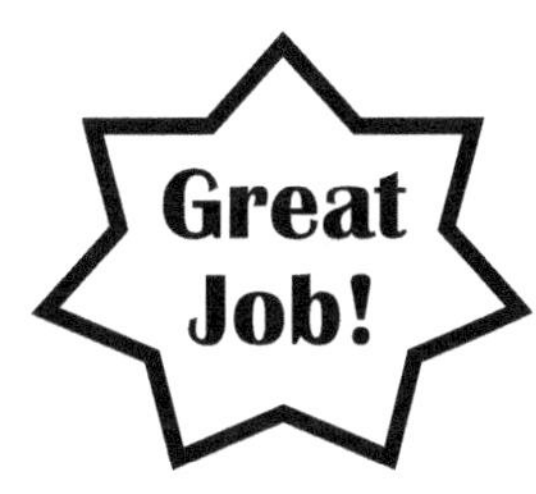

Throughout the book, I will make reference to your primary reason for exploring yoga. You'll want a handy reference to it, so either earmark this chapter, or better yet, jot down your written goal statement and empowering beliefs on a notecard to use as a bookmark. Keeping your eye on the prize of what you are trying to achieve will keep you motivated as we move through the rest of this book.

THE YOGI NEXT DOOR: MEET ALIA

Alia's first experience with yoga was soon after college. She was struggling with weight gain and looking for ways to incorporate exercise into her routine. Her mother had practiced yoga for as long as she could remember and thought that it might be a good fit for her. Intimidated by the idea of being the least flexible person in the room, Alia grabbed an equally uncoordinated friend and signed up for a local 12-week class. She was relieved to find that she felt like she belonged. "Along with traditional exercise," Alia says, "this [yoga class] was a critical piece of regaining my physical confidence and fitness."

When Alia got pregnant years later, she took prenatal classes. At that stage, she enjoyed the deep relaxation of prenatal yoga as well as the opportunity to meet a community of new moms. "I loved the way [prenatal yoga] made me feel. I slept so well after those classes!" Alia says.

Today, Alia practices Hatha Yoga once or twice a week. She finds that her practice has improved her balance and flexibility and allows her to start her day feeling calm, yet invigorated. For her, yoga is one part of her total fitness routine which includes strength training, cardio, and yoga. While she values all aspects of exercising, yoga was admittedly one part that she had not consistently practiced over the years, primarily due to budget constraints. In the past, she used her exercise budget to pay for a gym membership, which left her with little extra to pay for additional yoga classes. Thankfully, she recently found a gym that offers both under one membership. When asked what advice she would give to new students, she suggests a three-point plan:

1. Take a beginner's class,
2. Go with a light heart! It's OK to laugh, and
3. Go early and introduce yourself to the teacher and tell them you are new. You will get the most out of your class if your instructor knows how they can help you.

PART 2

WHAT IS YOGA?

Now that we've gotten over the hump of understanding why you're here and standing firm in your purpose for forging on, we can turn to the topic of yoga itself. There are many preconceived notions about what happens in a yoga class and what "type" of people practice yoga. **The main idea here is to get you more comfortable with yoga by providing some education and a common starting point.**

If intimidation by the unknown is part of what keeps you at bay, then this chapter should allay many, if not most, of your fears. For those of you who already have some yoga experience, I expect this section will help you make sense of those experiences in a way that you might not have understood previously, while also opening the door to further curiosity.

In Chapter 3, we will give a bird's-eye view of the history of yoga. Because yoga is an ancient practice, there is a lot that could be said. I have done my best to distill the highlights that I think are most relevant to a beginning student. Feel free to skip this chapter if you have some experience or a basic understanding of where yoga comes from.

In Chapter 4, we review in greater detail the many styles of practice you can find in the United States. I find that new students are often stuck when deciding what class to attend because they are unfamiliar with the styles and the language used to describe them. The discussion of the styles in this chapter will arm you with the necessary knowledge to navigate a schedule of yoga classes.

Chapter 5 will give you a better sense of what happens in a yoga class, as well as a discussion of certain variables that can impact your experience, such as the teacher, the environment, the community and the cost. This chapter will serve to set your expectations and drive your research process to find a good fit for you.

I know you're excited to move on, but first, a word about the use of Sanskrit in this text. Sanskrit is an ancient language that originated in India. The primary texts from which we have learned the techniques of yoga are written in Sanskrit. I've chosen to use both Sanskrit and English so that this book exposes you to language you might encounter on your own journey. Please do not let the Sanskrit frustrate or distract you. I will always provide both, so you can ignore the Sanskrit if you wish.

Chapter 3

A Brief Overview

The subject of yoga is extremely broad. For the purposes of this book, we just need to give you the basic picture of what yoga is and where it came from. I think it will suffice to paint a picture using broad strokes.

What is yoga? How do we begin to explain it? It is common to understand yoga as the practice of physical postures. As it turns out, yoga is much more than that! There are two distinct aspects to yoga: the techniques and the philosophy. You can take one without the other. They need not be practiced together, although they often are. It deserves emphasis here that while yoga does have a philosophy component, it is not a religion. The techniques and the philosophy are compatible with all religious faiths.

While there are these two parts to the practice, this book will focus primarily on the physical techniques. As you deepen your practice, you may consider pursuing a greater understanding of some of the other aspects. The practice of yoga prompts us to turn inward, bringing a greater awareness of our body, our breath, and our thoughts. We become curious about the other non-physical techniques. **The Sanskrit word "yoga" actually means "union," and represents bringing together the mind, the body and the soul.** As you continue with yoga, you will notice this integration and heightened level of awareness.

THE YOGA SUTRAS AND THE EIGHT LIMBS OF YOGA

The practice of yoga began a really long time ago in northern India. We're talking thousands of years ago, somewhere on the order of 5,000+[13] years ago. Originally, these practices were an oral tradition. People would pass the information down through generations by word of mouth. Sometime during the second century, a man named Patanjali noticed there was a system to these practices and decided to write it all down. We say that Patanjali "codified the principles of yoga," which means he catalogued them in an organized way. He did not invent the system of yoga, but he is certainly credited as the first person to record it. Patanjali's writings are compiled in a book called *The Yoga Sutras*.

***The Yoga Sutras* tell us there are eight aspects, or techniques, of a yoga practice that lead progressively towards the highest states of awareness.** In English, we refer to these eight steps as the Eight Limbs of Yoga[14]. In Sanskrit, you will hear the Eight Limbs referred to as "Ashtanga". Each of the eight limbs represents a distinct aspect of the yoga practice. The first four limbs refer to the physical techniques and ethical practices, while the second four limbs refer to meditation techniques.

While the system leads towards the highest states of awareness in a progressive way, it is not a distinctly sequential path. Most of us begin yoga by practicing the postures, even though it is listed as the third "limb" or step. As our practice progresses, aspects of other "limbs" may be introduced. Instead of moving from one step to the next, the path is more cyclical. Keep this in mind as we discuss the limbs in further detail.

THE FIRST TWO LIMBS: BEHAVIORS AND HABITS

The first four limbs of Patanjali's eight-fold path toward enlightenment address the gross, or outer body, preparing the body for the stillness of meditation and the free flow of the breath, or life energy.

The first two limbs are the social and behavioral guidelines—personal disciplines that can make our human experience more harmonious and joyful. They are often discussed in tandem. These guidelines are each observed, or practiced, mentally (thought), verbally (word), and physically (actions).

There are full texts devoted to explaining and analyzing these behavioral guidelines. Please don't get hung up on the details, as the meaning of each is not important at this point in your journey. I've included them here so you can have a sense of the whole system to refer back to when you're ready to learn more. The observance of the combination of both of these sets of guidelines might be described as "living your Yoga" or "a Yogic way of life". Appendix C has a table describing these guidelines in more detail.

THE THIRD LIMB: THE POSES

The third section of the eight-fold path references the poses themselves—the postures we practice in a yoga class. As suggested in *The Yoga Sutra*, the poses are intended to be held with stability and ease while regulating the breath. There are around 84 poses that are considered to be classical yoga poses.

THE FOURTH LIMB: BREATH CONTROL

Breath is life, and we learn that the ability to control the breath can alter our experience of any given situation.

Breath control practices are techniques to regulate the breath. What does this mean? It means we learn to take control of our breathing by adjusting its depth and length, which impacts the quality of the breath. We learn that, by controlling the breath, we can change the way we feel. There are many breath control techniques. One example is the Box Breath, and instructions for it can be found in Appendix B.

THE SECOND FOUR LIMBS

As we gain control of our behaviors, our bodies, and our breath using the techniques of the first four limbs, we learn to balance the energies that cause restlessness of the mind. This prepares us for the mindfulness practices of the next four limbs. These practices address the mind, or the inner realm, seeking to find a quieting of the mind that leads towards inner peace[15].

YOGA TODAY

Now that we know a bit about where yoga comes from, its ancient roots, and the basis for the modern practice, how does that translate to yoga today? Let me begin by telling you a story.

A few years ago, I went to an exhibit in San Francisco at the Asian Art Museum that was called "Yoga: The Art of Transformation". It was fascinating to learn that much of the early representation of yoga in the West was from photographs sent home from India by travelers, and later, those participating as contortionists in sideshows of the 1800s.

There were some crazy videos and photographs at the exhibit. The images of entangled and contorted bodies sent home on postcards were beyond anything I've ever seen in a yoga class. While Patanjali had already codified the practices of yoga in all eight of the limbs, it was the poses themselves that got the attention of the West. Even today, the postures are thought of as synonymous with yoga.

You will definitely encounter the poses in a yoga class, but you might also find exposure to the breathing practices and mindfulness techniques of the second four limbs. Depending on the teacher and the style, these other aspects may be emphasized to different degrees. We will discuss various styles of yoga in the next chapter, which will help you further understand the nuances of each.

To summarize, the practice of yoga began in India centuries ago and incorporates elements of ethical and behavioral guidelines in addition to a physical practice of postures, breath control and mind control techniques that lead toward unity of mind, body and spirit. Today, a yoga class in the Western world is usually limited to teaching the physical postures, but in a wide range of styles.

As we bring this chapter to a close, let me highlight the key concept I want you to remember: **yoga is more than just the postures!** Yoga is an eight-fold path called the Eight Limbs of Yoga, of which the postures are only one part. It just so happens that our yoga classes here in the U.S. tend to be primarily focused on the postures.

There are many different styles of practicing yoga, each with their own emphasis. The next chapter will introduce you to some of the most common styles that we practice in the United States, where they come from, and what you can expect from a class of each.

Remember, the path of a new yoga student can take more than one route. The entry point is typically the postures, with interest expanding into the other areas at one's own discretion, or based on the style of choice. If you are fascinated by The Eight Limbs of Yoga and the subtlety of the practice, you might consider seeking out further resources. I would suggest *The Spiritual Science of Kriya Yoga* by Goswami Kriyananda as a good place to start.

KEY POINT!

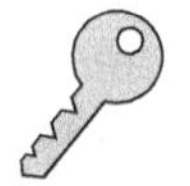

Yoga is more than just the postures! It is an eight-fold path, called the Eight Limbs of Yoga, of which the postures are only one part and the most common starting point.

THE YOGI NEXT DOOR: MEET JEREMY

After the birth of his first child, Jeremy found himself gaining weight. In his own words, "I had a baby and got fat." This realization motivated him to take up running and try a popular in-home exercise regimen called P90X, which offers daily videos to guide your workouts. In P90X, one day per week is devoted to yoga.

Jeremy says that he was surprised that he liked the yoga video as much as he did, given its length (90 minutes) and degree of difficulty. He describes it as his favorite workout as well as the most rewarding. With this regimen of running and P90X, Jeremy lost 60-70 pounds and was well on his way to being in the best shape of his life.

Knowing that Jeremy was enjoying the yoga portion of P90X, a friend invited him to an outdoor sunset yoga class on a nearby Lake Michigan beach. "I was hooked after that first one," Jeremy explains. "I loved how relaxed I felt afterwards." Attending the sunset classes made him realize that the P90X yoga experience was designed as more of a workout version of yoga. He was missing some of the more subtle meditative aspects of the practice, like the attention to the breath. Today, Jeremy continues his practice through the Ultimate Yogi Series on video as well as weekly sunset yoga classes in the summer.

When asked what kind of advice he would give to new students, Jeremy says, "Don't be afraid to fail, look silly, or go into child's pose. It's a personal journey, not a competition. Also, it's not just a workout. Find a good teacher who improves your mental state each class. You should leave with a smile, feeling renewed."

Chapter 4

The Many Styles of Yoga

Now that we know a bit about where yoga comes from and what it is, we can turn our attention to how it is practiced today. Below, you will find descriptions of the various styles of yoga commonly found in communities across the United States. I characterize these styles in a way that is both influenced by my experience and based on my own study. My intention here is to help you navigate a yoga studio schedule. One of the easiest hurdles to get over is simply understanding the labels and learning what the different stylistic names mean.

HATHA

If you learned anything from the last chapter, I hope you picked up that yoga classes, as we know them, are largely focused on the poses. This is important! **Hatha Yoga is an umbrella term for all the classical yoga postures**. The word itself is translated as "ha" meaning "sun" and "tha" meaning "moon", representing a balancing and uniting of opposites. Likewise, students should expect a Hatha Yoga class to be well balanced, with both standing and seated postures and a variety of forward folds, gentle backbends, and twists.

HATHA YOGA is a general term, used to describe physical yoga practice including postures and breathing techniques.

Aside from being balanced in this way, "Hatha" does not carry any other meaning or description of what you might expect from a class. It simply means the classical yoga postures will be practiced in whatever format the teacher chooses. A Hatha class is not branded and conforms to the teacher's unique style.

In a group Hatha Yoga class at our studio in Oak Park, the sequencing and presentation of the postures is open to the creativity of the teacher. Some teachers may incorporate breathing and meditation techniques. The level of intensity of our Hatha classes varies significantly based on the teacher. We have one teacher who leads a more fluid and invigorating class. By contrast, other teachers in our studio instruct longer holds and greater attention to the breath, without linking the poses from one to the next. Every teacher's style is their own, making each class a unique experience.

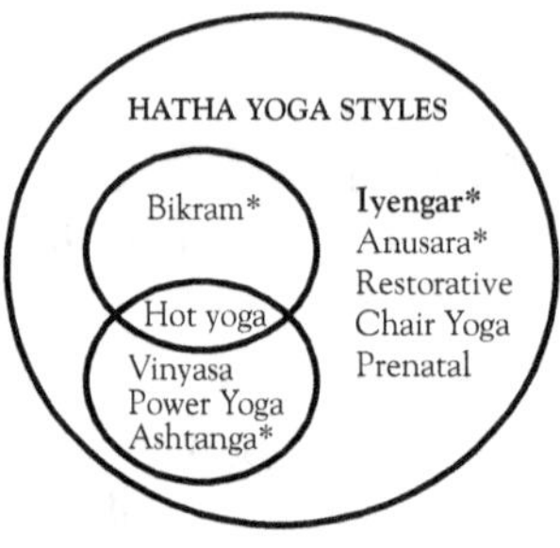

This graphic may help to explain the relationship between the different styles. Hatha encompasses everything. Vinyasa and Hot Yoga are two other broad delineators. The asterisks indicate branded styles, which means they have their own specific certification and the class experiences will be more standardized.

RESTORATIVE

The purpose of a restorative class is to deeply relax to the point of relieving muscle tension. Restorative classes are very therapeutic, helping to relax the nervous system and to boost the body's immune system. Most of the poses practiced will be on the ground, fully supported by props, requiring very little, if any, muscular work. Likewise, it would be rare for there to be any standing postures. Usually students stay on the floor in restful poses the entire time.

Restorative Yoga is a therapeutic form of yoga designed for deep relaxation. Specific styles of Restorative Yoga are Yoga Nidra, Relax and Renew® and iRest.

Yoga Nidra is another form that falls into the general category of Restorative Yoga, but is distinguished by the teacher reading scripts that are intended to induce a "yogic sleep" in which the students are aware, but so deeply relaxed as to be close to a sleep state. There are a few specific teacher training programs that are based on restorative yoga, but with their own branding. These go by other names, such as Relax and Renew® and iRest®.

VINYASA

The Sanskrit word Vinyasa means "to connect." In this practice, the poses are connected from one to the next with fluid movement. Sometimes, a class of this nature will also be labeled "Flow Yoga", drawing attention to the moving nature of the practice. These types of classes require cardio, strength and stamina. At times, a Vinyasa Yoga class may also be practiced in artificially high temperatures (see Hot Yoga, below), although that is not assumed based on the Vinyasa label alone.

At the studio where I teach, we use Hatha Vinyasa as a label for our flow-based classes to signal that we incorporate both dynamic movement and alignment instruction. Any class with Vinyasa in the label will typically include warm-up sequences that are repeated from one class to the next. This is particularly helpful for new students, as repetition is the key to learning any new skill.

ASHTANGA

Developed by K. Pattabhi Jois, Ashtanga Yoga is a style of Vinyasa. It is a physically demanding, flow-based practice that follows specific sequences. There are six sequences, or series, that increase in difficulty. In the U.S., what we call "Power Yoga" is based on this system. In its pure form, an Ashtanga class is an athletic and disciplined practice requiring strength and stamina.

HOT YOGA

Any class labeled Hot Yoga indicates that the class will be practiced in a room with artificially high temperatures (upwards of 90 degrees F). This style is not recommended for anyone who is pregnant or at risk of cardiac events. In my experience, hot yoga is typically a flow-based or vinyasa practice. Expect to sweat and be sure to replenish with lots of water during and afterwards.

Why the heat? The theory behind this form of practice is to mimic the conditions of the original practitioners in India, where it would have been practiced in high heat. Some people believe that these conditions are particularly good for recovery from injury. A yoga teacher friend of mine claims that yoga in high heat allowed her to recover from a serious back injury. Similarly, Bikram Choudhury (more on his style below) is said to have recovered from a back injury using the specific sequence he patented in his form of yoga. With high heat, the connective tissue moves more easily; you can stretch farther and perhaps go deeper into poses than you would otherwise. The downside to this style is that your body is so warm that it allows you to potentially stretch more deeply than your body is ready for, which can cause serious discomfort (or worse) in the following days.

BIKRAM

One form of Hot Yoga that is branded as its own is Bikram Yoga. Named after Bikram Choudhury, an Indian yoga teacher, this type of yoga is a specific sequence of 26 poses practiced in high temperatures (104 degrees F). Because each class is the same every single time, no matter what studio you go to, this practice is helpful for new students looking for consistency. Repetition is key when learning something new and eliminating the element of surprise can be very helpful to some people. This form is not suitable for pregnant women or anyone with cardiac health risks due to the high temperatures.

CHAIR YOGA

Chair Yoga is Hatha Yoga performed with the use of a chair for additional support. The chair mitigates some of the balance and strength challenges that are associated with traditional yoga postures. Students get experience with the postures in a well supported environment. While this type of class is open to all abilities, it is particularly welcoming for people with disabilities or physical challenges of any kind. I recommend Chair Yoga as an excellent entry point to the practice. I have an aunt who started Chair Yoga while in her 60s. She loves it and recommends it to all of her friends.

IYENGAR

In many ways, B.K.S. Iyengar is the modern-day father of yoga. Only recently passing on from his mortal life in 2014, B.K.S. Iyengar was long considered to be the authority on yoga. His book, *Light on Yoga*, was an international bestseller and continues to be a key reference. His style of practice has an alignment focus, which means he very specifically laid out how the bones should be lined up in the fullest expression of the postures. In an effort to make the postures accessible for those who are not able to achieve them at first try, he developed ways of using props to allow students with various abilities and ranges of motion to practice the postures.

Iyengar Yoga is a strict form of practice. There is great attention to the details of the pose and the hold times are relatively long.

Certification in the Iyengar tradition is a very long process that includes time studying abroad with the Iyengar family. This form of certification gives a teacher qualifications that go well beyond our current minimum national standards as defined by The Yoga Alliance, the national certifying body of yoga teacher training programs.

ANUSARA

Anusara Yoga is a branded style of Hatha Yoga. Developed by John Friend, Anusara Yoga is an alignment-based system with a lighthearted, upbeat philosophy[16]. Each class includes a theme and featured "heart quality"[17]. With this heart-centered emphasis, Anusara classes are intended to feel playful and uplifting with the expression of the poses coming from within. Props are used to meet every student wherever they are.

PRENATAL

As its name suggests, Prenatal Yoga is for pregnant women. In this class, a qualified teacher will guide students through a practice that is safe for both mom and baby. Typically, this form of yoga focuses on building strength and flexibility for birth, as well as deep relaxation techniques for managing the physical challenges of pregnancy. When I teach prenatal yoga, I like to incorporate some discussion at the beginning of class with the purpose of creating community for the students. We talk about topics such as preparing for childbirth, techniques for relaxation, doulas and breastfeeding. I find this helps to connect the other moms through their common experiences and curiosities.

Many moms ask me when it is best to start Prenatal Yoga. If you have no experience with yoga and are pregnant, I would recommend starting with a Prenatal class. If you have some experience with yoga, you should be able to reasonably continue your regular class until the second trimester or at whatever point your belly begins to get in the way. Transitioning to a prenatal class will make sure you observe proper guidelines to keep both you and baby safe in class.

This type of class is also appropriate for new moms in the postnatal period who want to return to gentle activity. Attending a prenatal class after giving birth can be a very nice segue back into exercise. I always suggest checking with the instructor in advance just to be sure they agree their class is appropriate for postnatal moms.

I have found that Prenatal Yoga is a common entry point for students new to yoga. Once moms get far enough along in their pregnancy that exercise options are limited, seeking out Prenatal Yoga is pretty common. Then, having experienced benefits from the practice, they continue beyond pregnancy and explore other classes.

KIDS' YOGA

Introducing yoga to children is a wonderful gift. Classes geared towards children are usually structured around a special theme, including an age-appropriate story, song, or craft. If the class is not a drop-off class, it might be labeled something else, like "Mommy & Me Yoga" or "Toddler Time Yoga". "Family Yoga" usually means parent and child. Read descriptions carefully to understand the appropriate age range(s) and cost structure.

WHICH STYLE IS FOR YOU?

Having spent a lot of time talking about the different types of yoga classes you might encounter, it seems like the next step should be to choose the one you want to practice. Surprise! We're not going to do that yet. Hear me out.

First, style is not everything. A yoga teacher brings their own way of sharing the teachings with their students, which transcends whatever label is chosen for the class schedule. For me, this is what makes experiencing more than one teacher so important. More on this later, but hold on to that thought: **the quality and style of the teacher has more influence on the resulting experience than the style of the yoga itself.** The same labeled class with two different teachers could be very different from one another. Key Point! If you take one Vinyasa class and hate it, it doesn't mean you necessarily hate Vinyasa! It could be that you just did not resonate with the teacher. Arming yourself with information about different styles of yoga, even though they may be broad descriptions, will give you a little more insight into what to expect.

KEY POINT!

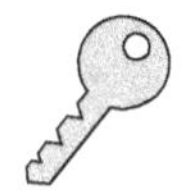

The teacher can have more influence on your experience than the style of practice.
If you don't like it, try a different teacher!

Second, we want to remain open to what's available. In Chapter 6, we'll begin researching classes in your area. You'll see that we'll start by looking for recommendations and then scanning the internet for supporting information on those classes, as well as other options near you. Likewise, we want to remain open to the available options, rather than dismissing something right now, just because the description here didn't speak to you. So we'll move on with an open mind and a wonderful reference in our hand to turn back to. Ready? Let's turn the page.

Bryan was first introduced to yoga at a boutique-style studio near his home. His wife asked him to join her a few times, so he somewhat reluctantly went to some Hatha Yoga classes there. He was one of the only guys in the class and always felt a little out of place.

A few years later, Bryan's boss invited him and some other coworkers to go with him do his daily Vinyasa Yoga class over their lunch break. Though he was skeptical, Bryan went along based on the promise of a great workout.

This second experience with yoga, Bryan reports, "was a totally different environment." The class was hot yoga, where yoga is practiced in elevated temperatures. He loved the Vinyasa style for the combination of strength, flexibility, and cardio. "If you're going to do one thing," Bryan says, "Vinyasa yoga hits everything."

From that first class, he was hooked. "That feeling when you leave the studio is amazing." From then on, Bryan and his co-workers would go to class three to four times a week.

Today, Bryan notices that his practice helps him to maintain strength and flexibility in his hip, which he injured a few years ago (Bryan suffered a hip dislocation and fracture). There are few activities that can do that for him.

About his experience with Vinyasa, Bryan says, "At first, you don't know the names of poses, you're watching the teacher or the students around you to know what to do, and you feel like you're constantly behind, trying to keep up. And then after a few classes, you get it and fall in to a routine with the instructor."

Bryan's advice for new students? "Ask a friend to go with you for accountability. I probably never would have practiced as much without someone to go with at first. And as you become a regular practitioner, I recommend changing it up–attend different classes and different teachers to keep things interesting."

Chapter 5
What to Expect from Class

There are certain things that you can expect from any yoga class—the flow of the class will follow a general pattern, as will the variety of poses that are covered. In this chapter, we will first review two aspects: the class structure and the individual elements of a well-rounded practice. In addition to the style of the class, which we discussed in Chapter 4, other factors that influence the experience of a yoga class are the teacher, the community, and the environment. These factors are less predictable, yet contribute to creating a unique experience. If you're looking for an idea of what to expect, this will give you a great start. Using the note-taking prompts, we will begin to keep track of any special needs or particular areas of concern you might have so we don't lose sight of them when we move towards researching classes in the next chapter.

CLASS STRUCTURE

The general arc of a yoga class is similar to any other form of fitness class: warm-up, the main body of the class, and a cooldown. Breaking that down further, I would say there are six parts of a yoga class: centering, warm-up, body of the class, cooldown, final rest, and closing. The combination of the style of the class and the teacher will dictate the poses and the pace, but this arc of the experience will generally stay the same.

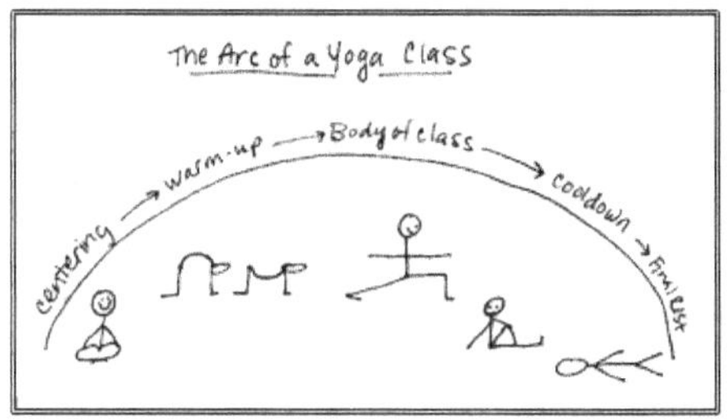

Centering

At the beginning of class, the teacher will usually ask the students to take a centering pose. This could be seated, standing, or lying down. It is a chance for the students to bring their focus inward and let the mind slow down, releasing what it took for them to get to class as well as thoughts about what is happening afterwards. Bringing awareness into the room and to one's breath are typical prompts from the teacher in the first moments of class.

In some cases, the teacher will ask the students to chant together the sound of "Om" (pronounced "aum"). This sound is a mantra, or vibration, that is traditionally chanted at the beginning and end of yoga sessions. It is said to be the sound of the universe. The purpose of making the sound can be as simple as helping to focus your awareness on the self. There is a long history and deeper explanation of this sound, but for beginners, suffice it to say that it allows you to turn inward.

Participating in making the sound is not required. Everyone's eyes are usually closed and no one will know if you've done it or not. You can skip it if it makes you uncomfortable or challenge yourself to do it if you are looking to stretch your comfort zone.

The teacher may also ask the students to choose an intention for their practice. This is something that took a long time for me, as a student, to get a handle on. When confronted with this request in class, a panic would come over me, not knowing what I should be paying attention to or choosing to focus on. If the teacher gave an example or two, I would usually take one of theirs.

In my opinion, the purpose of asking the students to do this is to help them focus their attention on their practice, full stop. As a new student, you are trying to integrate so much information that also choosing an intention can be overwhelming. If it causes you stress, as it did for me in my early years, you might choose for your intention to simply be for you to participate in the class.

It is important to point out that these aspects of the class I'm describing are not necessarily distinct. The teacher will not alert you as to when you're moving from the warm-up to the body of the class and so on.

Warm-Up

Every teacher has their own way of beginning a class. The intention of the warm-up is to bring greater circulation and to physically warm the body through movement and active stretching in order to prevent injury during the body of the class, where the majority of the work will be done. The style of the class will dictate what constitutes warming up. One suggestion is to warm up a little on your own before coming to class, particularly if you've never experienced the class before. Simply walking for five minutes before arrival will get your juices flowing and give you a head start.

YOGA HACK

Begin your warm-up by walking to class.
Park a few blocks away and use the extra steps.

Body of the Class

The body of the class will be the main emphasis of the class, perhaps taking up the majority of the time allotted. With the exception of Restorative classes, this is where a lot of the active stretching and strengthening will occur.

Cooldown

The class begins to wind down when the students come down to their mat for seated or supine (i.e., reclined) poses, oftentimes including postures designed to cool the body down (e.g., forward folding, twisting and some gentle backbends). Class begins to come to a close when the teacher brings the students down to the mat to wind down towards the final resting pose.

Final Resting Pose

The traditional final resting pose in a yoga class is called Corpse Pose ("Savasana"). For this pose, the students are lying down on their backs with the shoulders externally rotated so that the palms face up. The arms are moved slightly away from the body so air can circulate up into the armpits, and you allow the feet to splay outward. You softly close the

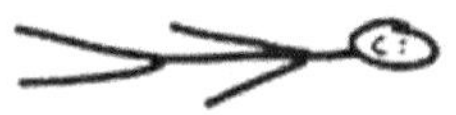

eyes and relax the throat, the tongue, and the soft palate in an attempt to relax the whole body, right down to the internal organs.

The teacher will prompt you through a series of cues to help you release all muscular work and allow your body to rest. Many people say this pose is the most important of the entire practice, since releasing muscle tension is one of the main purposes of the practice.

To come out of the final resting pose, the teacher will slowly bring your awareness back into the room and prompt you to make slow movements with your fingers and toes to bring energy back into your body. Then you bend the legs and roll to your right side. Turning to the right is intentional for purposes of sound digestion. Laying on your right side feels best. If you are pregnant, you will take Corpse Pose ("Savanasa") lying on your left side, in order to avoid putting pressure on the important vein that runs along the right side of your body.

Closing

To close a practice, the students move slowly to a comfortable, seated position. The hands are brought together in front of the heart center in prayer position. The teacher will say the Sanskrit word "Namaste" and the students respond with the same.

The word "Namaste" has deep meaning. Its direct translation is "I bow to you." When I teach, I often provide the following translation. "The divinity within me bows to the divinity within each of you." In our Kids' Yoga class, the teachers sing with the children this translation. "My little light bows to your little light. Your little light. Your little light. My little light bows to your little light. Na-Ma-Ste". I love that explanation, as it evokes the flicker of light of each of our souls, acknowledging the little souls of each other. Sometimes a teacher will also close with the sound of "Om," or some other chant.

Namaste is a Sanskrit word that is said at the end of a yoga class by the yoga teacher and then repeated back by the students. The word has deep meaning and is translated as "I bow to you". It symbolizes an acknowledgement of the Divine in each of us.

ELEMENTS OF A WELL-ROUNDED PRACTICE

A well-rounded yoga practice includes specific functional movements of the spine and limbs. A good teacher will be sure to incorporate each of them over the course of the class. There are a variety of ways to meet these requirements. In Appendix A, I explain each functional movement of the spine and limbs and give some examples of poses that create them. The main point is that **a variety of poses will be presented in a class setting, and in order for it to be a well-rounded practice, the poses will cover all movements of the spine and limbs**. You might also retain this idea for later, when I present some options for practicing at home.

KEY POINT!

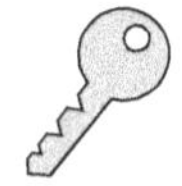

A well-rounded yoga class includes all movements
of the spine and limbs.

THE UNKNOWN

So far, we've covered the predictable variables of a yoga class: the arc of the class and the elements of a well-rounded practice. Now you can enter a class and reasonably expect the class to follow a general pattern with a sense of the motions that will be included. Clearly, the part that is more difficult to plan for are the unknown variables: the teacher, the environment, and the community. Each of these components can have a profound impact on the experience. Let's take a closer look at each.

TEACHER

Quite possibly the greatest influence on a student's experience, the quality of the teacher can overcome any number of shortcomings in other areas. **If you resonate with the teacher, you will want to go back.** Personality can play a big part here, but so can the quality of their voice, the vocabulary they use, or the life experience they bring to the practice. The brand of the studio or establishment hosting the classes might be what draws students in, but the majority of the time, the teacher will keep them coming back.

Vocabulary is one thing that plays a much larger role than people think. Depending on the audience, the analogies and references a teacher uses can

KEY POINT!

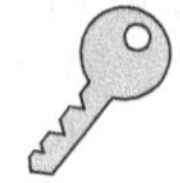

If you resonate with the teacher,
you will want to go back.

either get to the heart of their message or go way over somebody's head. Say, for example, there is a teacher that uses an extensive anatomy vocabulary. While the teaching may be accurate, the average beginning student might feel lost by the choice of terms and likewise be put off by the practice itself. This teacher will likely be better received by a group of medical and nursing students at a university hospital gym, rather than at their local community center.

And then there is something as simple as voice. We have a male teacher at our studio whose voice is so soothing that it almost doesn't matter what he says. The intonation of his voice ends up being calming and setting the tone in a way that allows the student's mind to relax and get lost in his words—a sort of meditation in itself.

You may find that some teachers will offer hands-on adjustments and assists, which is when a teacher mindfully places their hands on a student in an effort to guide the student's pose in a certain direction, to get them to go deeper into the pose, or to encourage a sensation that might be missing. A teacher should always ask permission before touching a student, even if they've known the student for a long time. Of course, teachers are also taught the appropriate way to touch so as to be respectful of a student's personal space.

Physical adjustments are a great way to deepen a pose and gain access to the pose in a way that was previously unavailable to you. As a student, I do like to receive adjustments from an experienced teacher and I also appreciate it when they ask for my permission. However, some people prefer not to be touched for various reasons and that's fine too. It does not detract from their experience at all.

The teacher and the traits they bring to a class can both attract and repel students. This is why I said earlier that the quality and style of the teacher has more influence on the resulting experience than the style of the yoga or any other factors. If you don't enjoy the class, but the location or environment is perfect, don't assume you hate the place or the style. Pay attention to what you liked and didn't like and try another teacher. I cannot stress enough the importance of trial and error in finding the right teacher for you.

YOGA HACK

If you don't enjoy a class, try a different teacher!
It may take some trial and error before you
find the right teacher for you.

ENVIRONMENT

Yoga classes are held in any number of spaces. Common places to find classes are dedicated yoga studios, gyms and community centers. Most of the time, you'll find these spaces to be soothing, with soft lighting and music playing in the background. However, the use of music, the presence of mirrors and props, the maintenance conditions and ambient noise are all things that can vary greatly from one class environment to the next.

Once you start looking, you will find every size of yoga space under the sun! When I lived in Baltimore, we lived downtown in one of the historical neighborhoods called Canton, right next to Fells Point. All the houses in this area are super narrow (as small as 12.5 feet across). One of the first yoga classes I went to in Baltimore was in the upstairs of an artsy retail space, in one of these narrow row homes. The mood of the room was very sweet with low lighting, hardwood floors, and light, flowing curtains. I happened to know the teacher from years ago as a camp counselor, which was a very nice surprise. There was only room in this studio for five mats; it was the smallest studio space I've ever experienced. It was very intimate, quite lovely for practicing, and only five students could participate.

On the other end of the spectrum, there are also very large spaces for yoga. My sister lives in San Francisco and often tells of going to classes with 100+ people in the room. She loves it—she follows a certain teacher all over town, no matter the circumstances.

I once taught in a large space, but with far fewer participants. It's an odd story. One of my friends in Baltimore was working at the FDA in Beltsville, MD. She was just starting to teach yoga and had gathered a small group of coworkers who wanted to practice after work once per week. There was one time when she needed a sub, so I taught for her. It was the very first class I ever taught! It was held in the lobby of one of the FDA buildings. The floors were carpeted and there was a decent amount of natural light with an atrium. I would not say it was lovely, but it was a nice atmosphere, albeit not private, and certainly convenient for those students. We had a nice practice there. If the size of the room or the number of participants matters to you, you might write that down for your list of research questions.

> What size class would you like to find?
> __Small (0-10 students), __Medium (10-30 students) __Large (30+)

The studio I teach at is on the bottom floor of a small apartment building. The tenant in the apartment immediately above the studio has recently changed and there is now a music teacher living there. When I teach evening yoga classes, it is common for us to hear the music teacher accompanying a student on the piano. Thankfully, she is a voice teacher and we mostly hear the lovely sound of her piano. We also often hear buses idling across the street or trucks pulling in to the grocery store to make a delivery. As a student, the ambient noise can be used as a tool to stay focused. Allowing yourself to be drawn to sounds wherever they come from is an opportunity to be present in the moment.

YOGA HACK

Use the ambient noise as a tool to focus your attention on the present moment.

In my conversations with new students, I have noticed that the topic of mirrors comes up quite a bit. As a teacher, I like to use mirrors as a helpful guide for students to check their own alignment, which helps keep them safe in class and teaches greater body awareness. Being able to see that your hips are in line with your heels or your knee is not extending beyond your ankle provides meaningful feedback to the student, as it can be hard to know where your body is in space without the use of the mirrors. However, I am also conscious of the fact that mirrors can cause anxiety for some students. The distraction of feeling exposed or looking at oneself or others can be debilitating. The good news is that there are plenty of places to practice that do not use mirrors or have the ability to cover them up (like we do in the space where I teach). If the idea of mirrors is a trigger for you, then acknowledging it is the first step to finding the right place for you to practice. If you think you would prefer for there to be no mirrors, then make a note of it here and be sure to ask about it when you research a class.

Will the presence or use of mirrors dissuade you
from going to a yoga class? __Yes ___No

If the answer is YES, aim to find a space that doesn't have them. ☺

Did you know that not all teachers use music during class? Most of the time, I teach without music. Honestly, this is mostly because I am lazy. I do not listen to music regularly and the idea of finding the right music to put together a playlist for my class seems tiresome to me. From a teaching perspective, I think it is a good exercise for students to be with their own thoughts, observing where their mind takes them in the absence of tone-setting music. This is where the opportunity of following ambient noise comes in. As a student, however, it does feel nice to walk in and have the tone set for the space with music. I do both, although usually I avoid the use of music.

When classes are held in yoga studios or gyms, it is common for all props to be provided, though sometimes for a fee. This may not always be the case, so I would add it to your list of things to ask about when you start researching classes. Are mats provided? Is there a cost associated with using them? The condition and maintenance of the props is something you may want to

Do you plan to use your own mat? __Yes ___No

If the answer is NO, be sure to ask if mats and other props
available and if there is a fee for use.

inspect before committing to using them. Your face, hands and feet may all end up in contact with a mat. Plan to bring your own if you have any issues with using a community mat.

COMMUNITY

The culture of the student community can certainly have an effect on the overall feeling of the place and its classes. Is the community small and tight knit? Or is it large and more anonymous? Which do you prefer? Does it matter to you?

At our studio, I am proud to say that we have a lovely community. The majority of our students consistently attend the same classes every week. Even though the classes are ongoing and advance registration is not required, the regularity of their attendance allows them to get to know one another. There is a feeling of camaraderie and it is welcoming.

Other studios or spaces may have a more anonymous feel. Remember my story about my sister in San Francisco who goes to classes with 100+ people in a huge room. She loves it. She may go with a friend, but she's not looking for community there. Both scenarios are fine. The question is, which one is for you? And maybe the answer is both! That's fine too.

Depending on the size, location and branding of the class, different target markets will be drawn to the class. Who attends classes at a certain location? Or at a certain time? There are likely to be differences in the crowd that attends classes in the early morning versus the middle of the day, versus the evening. When researching classes, you'll want to consider these factors. Are you interested in making friends with the students? Does it matter to you at all who is there? If so, ask some questions about the student base to get more comfortable joining them.

What type of community are you seeking?
___tight knit ___anonymous
___I'm not looking to make friends, but I'm open to it

What age range would you like for the students to be?
___around my age ___younger than me ___older than me
___age range doesn't matter to me

WHAT TO WEAR

The first thing to know about what to wear in a yoga class is that you will not wear socks or shoes. We practice yoga barefoot! The reason for this is so that you have good traction on the mat to prevent you from slipping. There are some sock-like products that are like gloves for your feet, with spaces for each toe and grips on the bottom. These are nice to use when you don't have a mat (in a hotel room, for example). If you are considering using them for sanitary reasons, I would advise buying your own mat instead.

What else to wear? Well, anything that will allow you to move freely and feel comfortable in your body. Whatever you normally exercise in is generally acceptable. The technology of high-performance fabrics is such that it is common for people to wear form-fitting clothes to class, but this is not necessary. It is most important for you to be able to move freely, being mindful that you would want your clothes to stay in place if you were to be partially upside down (as in touching your toes). Tucking in shirts and wearing sports bras are good ways to make sure you will not overexpose yourself if your outer layer is loose fitting.

The teacher in me would like to request that your knees be exposed so your teacher can see the alignment of the leg joints and bones (which will better allow them to keep you safe in class). The reality is that most people do wear pants to yoga class, although there are form-fitting pants that hug the leg in such a way that the knee is fully visible. When I attend class wearing pants that are loose through the leg, I roll them up so that my knee joints are exposed. I suggest you wear whatever is most comfortable for you. I know this is an area that can bring up body image issues, so I am sensitive that what to wear is not one size fits all.

YOGA HACK

What to wear to a yoga class:
1. No socks! Go barefoot
2. Unrestrictive, comfortable clothing
3. Preference for knees to be exposed or in fitted pants.

CHILDCARE

Yes, that's right, childcare! Some places have childcare on site. It's not always clear that this is an option, so it doesn't hurt to ask. At our studio, we are lucky to have childcare available (for only $3 an hour) and I think that it sets us apart from other local options. If you need childcare in order to carve out the time for formal yoga practice, and it is not available on site, I have some ideas for you. Check out Appendix D for some tips and tricks on the childcare dilemma.

YOGA HACK

Get creative with childcare for yoga classes by setting up swaps with friends. See Appendix D for details.

CLASS PRICES

There is a wide range of pricing for yoga experiences. I would say the cost for one yoga class averages anywhere from $10–$18. There will also typically be other pricing options that lower the per-class fee and encourage you to come back regularly. This may either be in the form of class packages (e.g., purchasing 10 classes for a 10% discount) or memberships (e.g., $90 for one month of unlimited classes). Look for expiration dates associated with all pricing options. In some cases, you will find discounts for students, seniors, and veterans.

Depending on your location and available offerings, you may also find classes that are discounted, free or donation only. These classes usually have different labels on a schedule, using terms like "Community Yoga" or "Donation Yoga". These words generally indicate that the class is offered at a reduced price ("Community Yoga") or at a price of your choosing ("Donation"). In the case of donation classes, they could be fundraisers (some or all of the collected funds are passed on to a charity) or simply that the clients pay whatever price they feel the class is worth to them. In either case, donation classes are not intended to be "cheaper" than the market rate, whereas the purpose of Community Yoga classes is to make yoga available to people in all circumstances.

If cost is a barrier for you, you might consider getting creative. After having visited a studio and paying for classes previously, approach the studio owner and ask if they have work/study programs. Assuming you have time to exchange for classes instead of money, this arrangement might work well for you. For example, at my studio, we have a front desk work/study position where a student comes in early to survey the studio for light maintenance needs and then handles the check-in procedures for the next two classes, attending one or both of them.

YOGA HACK

Save money by seeking out a work/study position where you offer your time doing administrative, marketing, or building maintenance in exchange for free classes.

Usually, these types of positions are not publicized. If this is something that interests you, I recommend checking the place out first before asking about the possibility of work/study. Determine if you like it there and then strike up a conversation about work/study. As an employee of sorts, it is really important that you have a desire to be there, that you like the atmosphere and could see yourself practicing there on a consistent basis. If you are committed to it, I am sure you could make something happen, even creating a position that didn't previously exist. In my experience as a director, these types of arrangements are completely individualized.

Yet another way to look at the expense is that you are worth it. So many of us get excited about investing in our home, our retirement, or our education, but forget that investing in our health and wellness has exponential returns as well. Are you in physical pain? Emotional pain? Remember those reasons that brought you here? We talked about them in the very first chapter and you came up with your own purpose. Pull out your notebook and take a look at the purpose you wrote down. That is the reason why investing in yourself makes sense and might take precedence over other aspects of your budget. Many of us live by default, rather than by design, and our spending habits show it. Make the shift to choose your destiny by carving out time and money for this important practice. Your health depends on it!

SPECIAL CONSIDERATIONS

I realize that this section on unknown variables is kind of funny to even include. There are as many variations here as I can imagine, so how can I prepare you for what to expect? The thing is, some of these things will make a profound difference. Also, I think it's important to emphasize that there is a wide range of variation. All kinds of people practice yoga in all kinds of places. Yoga class is not always practiced in the way you imagine it in your head. I'll say that again: **Yoga class is not always practiced in the way you imagine it in your head!** So many of us carry around an image or idea of who practices yoga, how it's done and where, and for every example that fits your mold, there are most certainly some that don't.

KEY POINT!

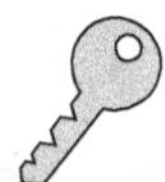

There are many different ways of practicing yoga—it may not be just like you've imagined!

So make a note for yourself here: what will you want to find out about a class before attending based on what we talked about in this chapter? Go through the Write It Down prompts and pull together any areas you'll want to cover in your research of classes. Are you interested to know about the size of the class? The general age of the students? The cost of the class? Will you need childcare? Do they have mats? This will be your start.

You'll also want to review Chapter 2 and your desired benefits from the practice. Remind yourself of what you'd like to gain from practicing yoga. Make a note of it along with the other special considerations so that you make sure to include it in your process of discovery.

Scan through this chapter and write down what is important to you in a new yoga experience, including the primary benefit that you seek from practicing.

In the next two chapters, we will pull together a list of places that offer yoga and evaluate them based on these questions you've just jotted down. Finding out more than just the time and place in advance can save you a trip if you know more about what kind of experience you are looking for. All these factors we've discussed in this chapter can make or break your experience. None of it is right or wrong, you'll just find that you like some classes and not others. **You will find a class that works for you.** You can do this!

THE YOGI NEXT DOOR: MEET MAUREEN

Maureen was first introduced to yoga by her mom. In her words, "I was in college in 1999 and I opened an envelope to find Xerox copies of an instructional manual of yoga poses. My mom had taken a few classes at the local park district and thought well enough of the experience that she found it worth sharing. Keep in mind, this meant borrowing the book from the teacher, going to the library to copy the pages, putting them in an envelope and mailing them a few states away." It was a big effort for her mom to do all of that, and the point was not lost on Maureen. She started doing the poses on her own and liked how they made her feel.

She didn't attend a class until several years later when her husband bought her a class package to a local studio. In those first few classes, Maureen felt a bit out of place. "I remember feeling hot with embarrassment at the end of [my first] yoga class where the instructor played chimes and asked us to say "Om". I thought, 'What cult have I joined?!' I was definitely uncomfortable and felt out of place.

While she was a bit uneasy, the physical conditioning and mental lift that she got from the practice was enough to keep her coming back. Eventually, after years of practice "without a single person asking her to join a séance", she relaxed and began to appreciate the more spiritual aspects of yoga. Today, she reports, "One of my favorite parts of class is lying down [in the final resting pose] while the rest of the class chants "Om" or singing bowls are played. The reverberations feel like tiny massages on my spine and the sounds are so satisfying."

Practicing three to four times a week, Maureen enjoys Vinyasa flow classes and says that she appreciates that yoga makes both her body and her mind stronger. The biggest benefit of her practice, though, is the mental clarity and stress relief. "When I have a busy day, I'm so tempted to skip yoga and give that hour to work or my family, " Maureen says, "But I have yet to regret going to a class. When I sit back down at my desk, I work without pressure or stress. I sit up straighter and I respond to emails and tasks with more clarity and less annoyance. I come home to my family lighter and with more ease. I have no doubt yoga makes me better at my job and better at relationships."

What are the keys to maintaining her strong interest? She reports that "euphoric is not an exaggeration" of how she feels at the end of most classes! A little bit of change helps too. When she travels for work, she gets the chance to visit new studios, new teachers and try new styles. After these new experiences, her regular classes seem fresh.

When asked what advice she has for new students, Maureen suggests, "Give yourself three months before deciding if it's right for you. Classes drastically vary by teacher and style and it can be frustrating when you don't know the poses and can't understand the Sanskrit [if it's used]. See if you feel better about life after three months, then decide." Further, she advises, "Yoga is a metaphor for leaps of faith. When I saw someone do a headstand for the first time in class, it struck me as otherworldly. Then I wanted to be otherworldly. So step by step, I learned how to build up to it and now when I'm overwhelmed or sad I stand on my head and for some reason the world improves."

PART 3

GETTING STARTED

Welcome to Part 3! You are halfway through your journey towards developing a yoga practice. We talked about what brought you here in Part 1 and set out some foundational knowledge and expectations about the practice in Part 2. In Part 3, we will roll up our sleeves and figure out how best to get you practicing. This is where you meet the yoga mat!

In my yoga teacher training, I was taught that the best way to get your point across to students is to tell them what you are going to tell them, tell it to them, and then tell them what you've told them. I'll follow that model here, by giving you an overview of what our strategy is to get you practicing and then give you the details of each part of that strategy in the following sections, followed by a summary at the end.

Our research process has three main aspects to it: Conversation, Research, and Experience. We begin with conversation: talking with friends, family and community. This gives you some context and a starting point. Talking with a friend about their own experience will hopefully shortcut your research process and add value quickly. Next, in the Research section, we will talk about how and where to look for classes, teachers, and yoga instruction resources, as well as further evaluate suggestions you may have gotten from other sources. In the Experience chapter, we will discuss your plan for getting some yoga experience before committing to a regular practice. Trying more than one class before choosing the best fit is often a wise move. When shopping for any major purchase, do you ever buy the first item you find? Not usually! This section will close with some guiding principles as you move toward a regular practice.

Chapter 6
Find Local Classes and Teachers

There are four main sources of information for finding in-person yoga classes: personal referrals, the internet, local publications and local gathering places. Let's look at each of them. I don't believe you need to explore all these avenues, but you do want to find a handful of classes that match your style, interest, and basic availability as far as location and logistics. We'll start a running list of places you find in the margin for later reference. Continue to follow the advice in this chapter until you've found up to a handful of good choices. If you happen to live in an area with only one or two options, that's Ok! We'll work with what you've got. I suggest exhausting the suggestions in this chapter to be sure to find obscure, lesser-known opportunities. I've offered these resources in order of priority. We'll start with personal recommendations and go from there.

YOGA HACK

How to find a yoga class, listed in order of priority:
1. Personal referrals
2. Internet searches
3. Local publications
4. Local gathering places

TALK WITH FRIENDS

When you are in search of a recommendation for the best burrito in town, a good car mechanic, or babysitter, whom do you talk to? Many of us have our go-to sources for such things. I use Angie's List for contractors and Yelp for restaurants. **But I almost always put more weight on a friend's recommendation than an outside source.** For this reason, I think it's best to start your research for yoga classes with family and friends.

By asking a few people about their experiences, you might be able to spend less time searching the internet or pounding the pavement. My husband has a friend who is known for exaggeration. If she were to tell me she went to a class that was so awful she had to walk out, I would probably assume it couldn't be that bad, simply because I know her and how she talks about things. By contrast, if I read that review online, I might completely discount the place because I don't know enough about the reviewer.

So which of your acquantainces should you ask about yoga? Everyone and anyone! For the next two days, make a point to tell everyone you come in contact with that you are interested in exploring yoga and taking a class. Cast this net wide: family, friends, neighbors, and coworkers. You'll probably be surprised by how much information you get this way and find that someone you know practices or has experience and you didn't even know it.

If you are not totally comfortable with everyone knowing about this search, then, of course, feel free to be modest about it. You might curate a list of people you would be comfortable approaching, which will do just fine. You do not need to go far out of your comfort zone for this one. You might find someone willing to invite you to practice with them, which can be a nice introduction and a great way for you to expand your relationship.

I know we're not all scientists here, but when you're doing research, you probably realize that a larger sample set is better than a smaller one, so speak with more than one person. **If you're having one-on-one conversations, shoot for at least two or three,** but know that five or ten is better! And check this out: you might learn something interesting about your friend that you wouldn't have known otherwise.

WHAT TO ASK

Next, the question is what to say? What information do you want? And how do you elicit that information? Here is a list of questions that will get you going. It's pretty thorough, so don't feel like you need to go through all of them, but these will definitely keep the conversation moving if your friend isn't quite sure what to tell you about their experiences.

YOGA HACK

Go to my website at
www.dianashea.com/readyforyoga to get
an interview template with these questions

---

1. Where do you practice? Or what resource do you use to practice? (not always in-person formats)
2. What teacher(s) do you recommend?
3. What style of yoga do you practice?
4. Why did you start practicing yoga?
5. What benefits do you see from your practice?
6. Why do you continue your practice?
7. Would you recommend the class you take? Why or why not?
8. What do you not like about the class?
9. Do you have any suggestions as I start my research? Where are some good places for me to look for classes in town?
10. Any other suggested resources?

> Start a list of classes, studios or teachers you want to follow up on based on your conversations and other research.

REFERRALS

Do you have an acupuncturist? A chiropractor? Or a massage therapist? These professionals commonly refer their patients to complimentary healing modalities, so they might have some suggestions for you. Are you a client of any professionals in the sample list below? If so, be sure to include them in your search for local yoga information. Ask for a referral to a good yoga teacher. They might know one.

- Acupuncturist
- Chiropractor
- Social worker (school, library, community center)
- Massage therapist
- Psychologist
- Life coach
- Midwife
- Naturopathic doctor

CROWDSOURCING

Speaking with friends and family one-on-one is a very good way to execute this conversation piece. Another way to get recommendations from your community is to crowdsource the information through a variety of means, like email and social media. Regarding your sample set, this method of getting recommendations will likely increase the number you get.

The most basic format would be to write an email describing your interest in beginning a yoga practice and seeking recommendations. Collect the email addresses of the friends you'd like to contact and send your template to each of them. This works well if you are contacting a small number of people or have your email addresses managed in a convenient way. You can write your own email or you can use the following sample as a starting point and adjust it as needed.

"Hi Friends,

I'd like to find a beginner yoga class with less than 10 students somewhere near my home. Do you have any recommendations? Or experience with beginning yoga classes? I've decided I want to work on quieting my mind and slowing my life down and I know this will be a good way for me to learn how to do that. Any advice you might have would be appreciated. Thank you!"

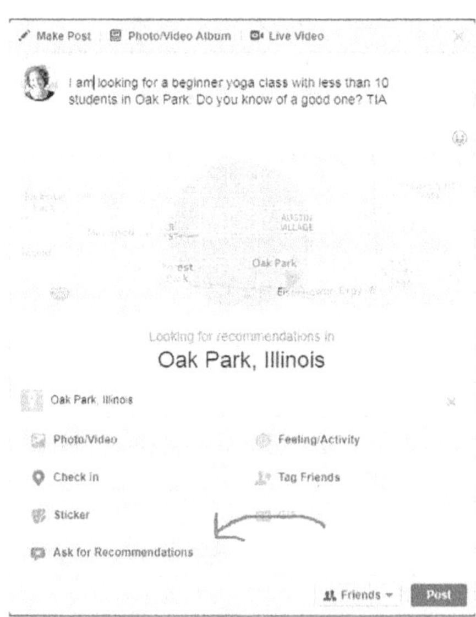

A popular format for polling larger numbers of people are social media platforms like **Facebook and Nextdoor**. Posting to your personal account or local group pages gives you the opportunity to seek information from your various communities. I'm part of a Facebook group for working moms who live in Oak Park, IL. This group is assumed to be busy and efficient with their time, so we frequently look to each other for recommendations for all kinds of things. Here is a sample post for Facebook. Use the "Ask for Recommendations" feature when posting in the status bar. Use your own motivation for practice to write a social media post looking for recommendations. A common abbreviation to indicate this type of post begins with ISO, which stands for "in search of".

After giving some time to accumulate responses, be sure to go through them and add to your list of classes, studios or teachers you want to follow up on. Hopefully you can lean on the experience of your network to come up with a few good suggestions.

BEWARE OF THE NEGATIVE BIAS

As you broaden your research to social media, you'll find a wide range of input. My final disclaimer on this is that there will always be a "negbomb" looking to drag you down. I'm sure I date myself by using that word. A negbomb is someone who uses their own misery to infect others with more misery. Furthermore, the negative bias of our brain chemistry can cause people to react more strongly to negative experiences than to equally positive experiences. Our brain latches on to negative comments, making it difficult to overcome them[1]. I believe the general belief is that it takes five positive reviews to outweigh a negative one. Bottom line: if you post your questions to public, or even closed group arenas online, you are bound to get a decent number of negative reviews.

So how can you measure the usefulness of a negative post? Going beyond a star rating or thumbs up/thumbs down will help to better understand the pros and cons of an establishment. Be mindful of the content. Is the person lodging a specific complaint? Does the bad experience pertain to a specific teacher? Or to the studio/space? Does the comment lead you to believe you would be uncomfortable going there? Taking a deeper dive into the specifics of the reviews will help you to separate those one-off bad experiences from what might otherwise be a trend. I know this isn't the first time you'll have used online reviews—use your best judgement and place greater emphasis on personal recommendations.

GOOGLE

We all know that when looking for information on the internet, you can easily "google" it. This will bring up a wide net of results that vary significantly depending on your search terms. I would suggest starting with

"Yoga near me". This will bring up a list of businesses that self-identify as offering yoga classes, as long as Google has your correct location. Keep in mind it might not be an exhaustive list because some yoga studios are better than others at getting their listings included. Google also has user reviews, although their use varies greatly from market to market.

YOGA HACK

Begin your internet search for classes by googling the phrase "yoga near me" or "yoga near [insert address]".

YELP

Yelp markets itself as a directory. I see it as a user review and advertisement platform. A Yelp search will bring up any yoga Yelp pages in the area of your search. This search might produce a different result set than your Google search because of the rules around how a Yelp page is created and maintained. This tool can be quite helpful if you find places with reviews because you can see what some of the local thoughts are on the experience.

As a user, you can see how many reviews a user has written, which could help to substantiate their remarks. Yelp also filters the reviews using an algorithm (which I am not privy to). Certain reviews are not "recommended" by Yelp and are therefore not shown or taken into account when averaging the business' star rating. This is to protect both the business (from one-time negative reviewers) and the user (from one-time positive reviewers who may have an interest in the business). In general, it is difficult to weigh the validity of the reviews on an individual basis, so take them each with a grain of salt and look for trends in the comments. I would suggest starting by looking up the names of the places that have been most highly recommended based on your conversations and crowdsourcing. Read the reviews and decide if they should stay on your list of possibilities.

Remember to keep adding to your list of places to follow up with as you learn about them.

MINDBODY APP

When it comes to looking for yoga classes, there are some more directed resources that may increase your results. MindBody is an online software platform that many yoga and other fitness and wellness studios use for scheduling and registration. There is an accompanying free smartphone app that allows you to search anyone in their network for specific classes near 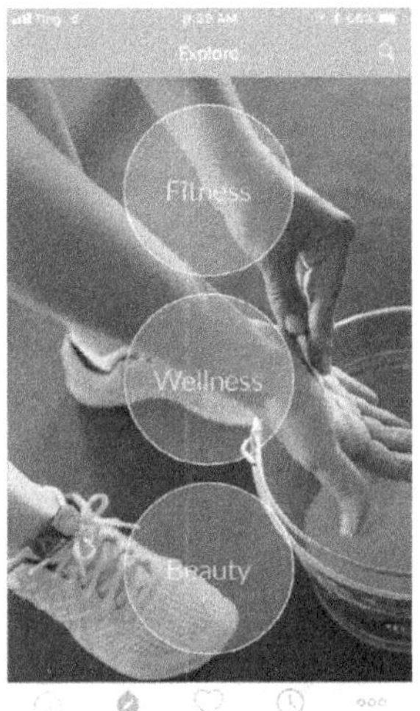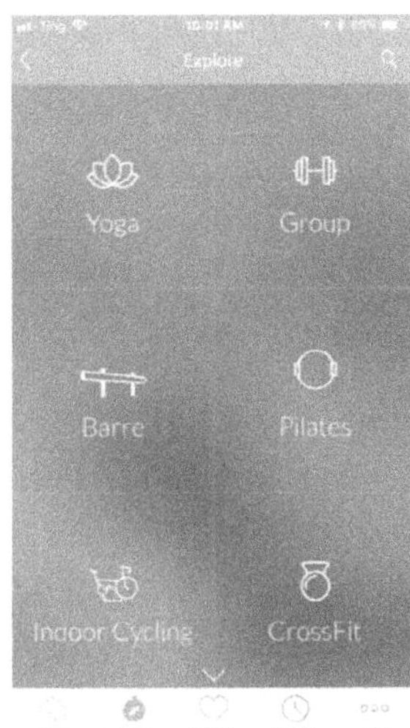 you. Really hear me on that one—**only those studios and teachers that use the MindBody app to handle their online scheduling will be found in the MindBody app.** This means that it is only a subset of all of the local possibilities. When you search, it will give you the time, place, and teacher all at once. You can even register for the class from the website or app itself. This can be used for yoga, but also for a range of other things like spinning or massage. The broad search categories are Fitness, Wellness and Beauty. After selecting Fitness, you drill down further into Yoga and then input your location. Download the app and check it out—it's pretty cool.

YOGA TRAIL

Yoga Trail (www.yogatrail.com) provides a combination of the features present in Yelp and MindBody, except it is only for yoga. It is a searchable directory of yoga teachers and places along with user reviews and class schedules.

When you log in to the site (it does require you to create a username and password before searching), you can enter your location and search for Classes, Events, Teachers or Places. With this function, it seems like it should be the best place to get information about local classes, but in my experience, it is incomplete. The studios and teachers are required to update their current

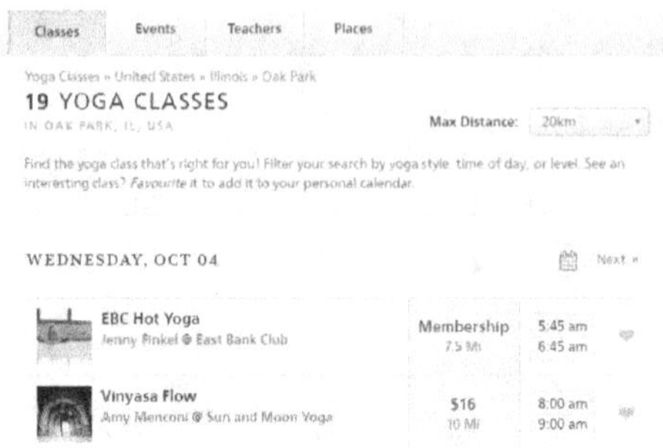

schedules on the Yoga Trail platform in order for them to be found in the results. In other words, Yoga Trail is not able to aggregate the data from other sources, but relies on the self-reporting of the yoga providers. I am sure the completeness of the information depends on the market.

I recommend using it to search for teachers and places and then doing further research on their respective websites. If you find a class schedule on Yoga Trail, please confirm its accuracy before clearing your calendar to attend!

YOGA ALLIANCE

The Yoga Alliance (www.yogaalliance.org) is the national certifying body for yoga teachers in the United States. It's a non-profit agency that supports the yoga industry through accreditation and continuing education. On their website, you can find a teacher, first by location, and then filtered by teaching designation, style and language spoken. The user can further sort the results based on distance, teaching hours, or name. **This site is particularly helpful if you are looking for information on a certain teacher because you can see where they teach and contact them accordingly.**

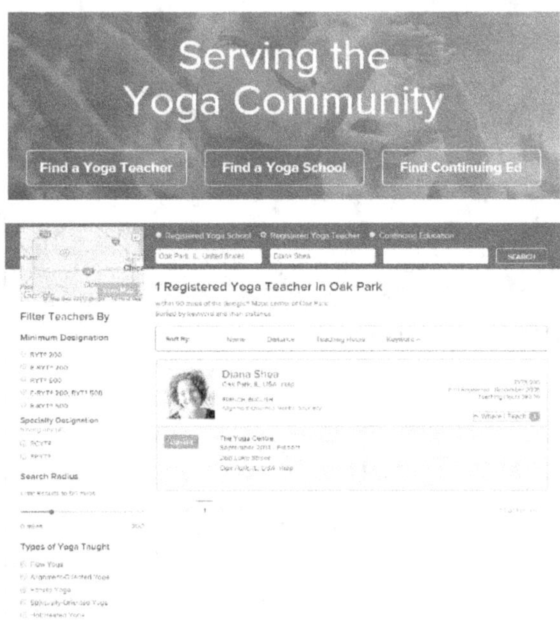

Understanding teaching credentials is important for your own safety. If you're reading this book, I'm going to guess you would not be able to distinguish a high-quality lineage of apprenticeship from a less impressive one. That's why the Yoga Alliance was created. It serves as the national certifying body for teacher training schools and standardizes the education of yoga teachers.

However, as with any profession, the teaching designation is only one piece of information you need to evaluate a teacher on paper and better understand their qualifications.

YOGA HACK

Looking for a certain teacher? Or specific style?
Use YogaAlliance.org to find classes near you
that meet your requirements.

There are four types of teaching designations that indicate a combination of the number of teacher training hours and the number of teaching hours completed by the teacher. They are as follows: RYT 200, E-RYT200, RYT 500, and E-RYT 500. There are two sequential levels of teacher trainings: 200 and 500. The designations that begin with "E" stand for "Experienced" and indicate a significant number of teaching hours. Appendix E gives greater detail on the teaching designations and their differences.

YOGA ALLIANCE TEACHING CREDENTIALS

1) RYT 200 - basic training
2) E-RYT 200 - basic training plus 1,000 teaching hours
3) RYT 500 - highest level of training
4) E-RYT 500 - highest level of training, plus 2,000 teaching hours

Remember to keep adding to your list!

LOCAL PUBLICATIONS

Between using the websites I've mentioned and talking to your friends, you should be able to come up with a quick list of yoga classes and places near you offering them. There are still a few other ways to find out about yoga classes that fall along more traditional lines and may even feel outdated. I have decided to mention them here in case you are a more hands-on person.

As I've mentioned before, I live in Oak Park, IL, which is 10 miles west of downtown Chicago. We have a few small, suburban newspapers that cater to this area. As the director of a local yoga studio, I submit information about our classes to these small papers to include in their local events or calendar sections. Does your town have something similar? If there is a wellness column or section of the paper, keep an eye on it to see if they ever highlight yoga.

If you live in a bigger city, you might also have access to publications with a category focus that would advertise yoga classes and events. Here in Chicago, we have three publications that come to mind: Yoga Chicago (www.YogaChicago.com), Natural Awakenings Chicago (http://www.nachicago.com/) and Illumine Chicago (www.illumineChicago.com). These are three go-to resources for all information regarding yoga classes or opportunities in and around the Chicago area.

Another angle is to look for publications that cater to specific demographics, like seniors or parents. For example, here in Chicago, we also have Chicago Parent (www.chicagoparent.com), which lists all kinds of opportunities for kids, parents, and families.

Do you have yoga-related magazines in your area? Or do you fall into a demographic that has its own publication? **If the market you live in is large enough, your area may have a publication that focuses on the category of yoga or a demographic that you identify with. Find it!**

LOCAL GATHERING PLACES

When you're out and about, can you think of any place that has a community bulletin board? Usually it has a bunch of flyers on it or stacks of business cards sitting out. Sometimes you don't even notice them, but they are typically in the back of the store by the bathrooms or near the front entrance. Start to think about your local coffee shop and library—do they have something like this? Mine do. **Here's a list of places I find generally have community boards where flyers for yoga classes are commonly posted:**

- health food stores
- vegetarian restaurants
- juice bars
- coffee shops
- food co-ops
- libraries

Pounding the pavement can be helpful when looking for information about local classes, but going straight to places that offer this type of programming is also a good idea. Do you spend any time at a fitness club? Does your city have a Parks and Recreation department? Or Senior Center? These can be good resources for information about local classes if you do not know where the classes might be offered. It is pretty common for yoga to be available in health clubs, parks and recreation buildings, and senior centers. If you have access to any of them, be sure to include them in your search. **Here is a list of common places that offer or host yoga classes:**

- Fitness clubs
- Yoga studios
- Senior centers
- Community colleges
- Colleges/Universities
- Park District / Parks and Recreation
- Athletic apparel stores (e.g., Lululemon)
- Chiropractor offices
- Integrative Medicine physician group offices

THE LIST

At this point, your list has surely grown. It includes your community recommendations as well as the places you've discovered through local research, either on the ground or online. Next, we'll move on to evaluating the choices and getting some experience! We're almost there.

Chapter 7

Evaluate and Experiment

Now that you've got your list in hand of possible places or teachers to meet, we'll figure out which ones to try. Getting exposure to some yoga is going to be the most informative part of this process. You can read about it until you are blue in the face, but until you get your body on a mat, you won't have the direct experience to inform you how best to proceed. This is it! We have arrived at our point of transition—it's time for you to take action.

So how do we move forward? Based on your desired benefit from the practice (from Chapter 2), what you know about the different styles of yoga (from Chapter 4), your preferences and curiosities (from Chapter 5), and your research (from Chapter 6), we will narrow your list. Ideally, you'll use this process to come up with a short list of three to five classes that you'd like to try and make a plan to visit one or two.

THE SHORT LIST

Do you remember in Chapter 5 when we talked about what to expect from class? I prompted you at the end of that chapter to jot down any areas that are important to you or that you might like to confirm before attending class. Go back to that page and review your comments. Using that list, you'll go to the relevant websites to glean more detail about the class offerings. You're looking for things like cost, class times, style names, and childcare (if you need it). Put in a phone call, if possible, to get more personalized information about the class. Start a worksheet that pulls together all your research and create a list of classes that includes information about the location, teacher, and style.

YOGA HACK

Download an evaluation template from my website:
www.dianashea.com/readyforyoga

Now it's time to make some choices. Based on what you know, highlight the classes you would be open to attending at least once. Did a friend recommend a class that would work for you? Highlight that one! Going with a friend can be a nice intro. Remember, we're only looking to get some experience and exposure under our belt. Forget about any limiting factors that would prevent you from making a commitment, we just want exposure at this point. If you find a great match right out of the gate, that would be great, but it's not required.

SCHEDULE TWO CLASSES

Take a look at your list. The highlighted classes comprise your short list. This is where the rubber meets the road (or your feet touch the mat)— excitement! Choose one class from your short list and schedule the time to go. Make whatever arrangements you need to clear your calendar at that time in the next week or two and attend the class. **I often tell students that the most difficult thing about practicing yoga is getting there!** Seriously! Setting the alarm to wake up early, or making dinner ahead of time so it's waiting for you when you get home, or clearing your work calendar so you can scoot out for a class right on time as you swat away co-workers—these are all tactics for evading the things that can easily distract or dissuade us from putting ourselves first and making sure we make an investment in our health.

So what do you need to do in order to make the time to attend that class? Look at your calendar and consider the details. Then reserve a space for yourself in the class if they take advance registration. Put it in your calendar or otherwise set a reminder for yourself.

I'll give you a minute. Come back when you've got that arranged.

KEY POINT!

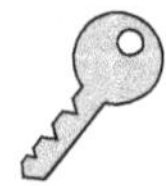

Oftentimes the most challenging part of a yoga class is just getting there.

Congratulations! You've scheduled your first yoga class and you're on the right path. Now let's choose the second class you'll attend. Wait, what?! I know, you thought you were done. When you are just starting out, I think it is a good idea to try at least two, preferably three classes before choosing one for a regular practice. However, if you feel good about the first class you attend, great. Go with that one and schedule it into your calendar for the next several weeks. If you don't happen to like the first class, it's a good idea to have a second class already planned. Now, go on and schedule it into your life, making whatever arrangements are necessary. I'll give you another minute.

Great! Now you're good to go. Take one last look at your short list and choose the third class you'll schedule.

EXPOSURE

Holy cow, we're finally here! You're going to a yoga class! Now it's time for me to step aside and let you go out there and get some exposure to yoga. I know you can do it. Give yourself an actual pat on the back for making it this far and stepping out to try!

Once you've gone to your first class, you can decide if you want to stick with that one or continue with the second or third that you've scheduled. As you get more experience, you'll be better able to compare and decide which will work best for you. We've done a lot of work here so you will know what to expect, but at the end of the day your gut (and your body) will tell you whether a class is right for you.

> For each class that you try, reflect on your experience by answering these questions. What did you like about the class experience? What part of the class experience could have been better for you? Would you like to go back? Why or why not?

If your first experience isn't what you hoped, fear not! That's why you have a second and third option lined up. A class might have checked all the boxes for you in advance, but when you got there it didn't seem quite right. That happens! Don't be discouraged. The point is to get your feet wet. Attending two to three different classes gives you some information about what it's like to practice yoga and perhaps some of its benefits you hadn't previously experienced.

Chapter 8

Guiding Principles for Your Practice

I have some guidelines I share with my own students, and I'd like to include them here. Having some guideposts to hold on to as you approach your practice will be helpful on this new journey. I also encourage you to go back to your notes from Chapter 2, where we explored your driving force for practicing yoga. You answered the following questions: Why are you interested in learning more about yoga? What would you like to gain from developing a yoga practice? How would your life be different if you practiced yoga? Reread your answers to these and keep them top of mind. Remember, keeping your eye on the prize of what you are trying to create will keep you motivated. It will also help you avoid discouragement.

EMPTY STOMACH

It is best to practice on an empty stomach (at least two hours after eating).

HYDRATE

Drink water throughout the day, even during class. Thirst is the first sign of dehydration, so it is important to support your body's normal functioning through regular hydration. Room temperature (or warmer) water is best because it is closest to your body temperature.

EVERY DAY, ANY AMOUNT

Any amount of yoga practice is worthwhile. If possible, practice every day, any amount.

SAFE JOINT ALIGNMENT

Hatha Yoga poses are designed to re-establish our body's intended skeletal alignment. Our bones are designed to bear the weight of the body. Thus,

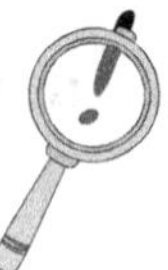

Correct **Joint Alignment** is important for avoiding injury, both from repeated stress on weaker parts of the joint and from acute incidences.

when they are aligned properly, the muscles have little or no work to do and can release their gripping or tension. Also, **observing correct alignment of the joints can help protect them from harm.** Use these tips, as well as the guidance of qualified teachers, to practice yoga safely.

KNEES

- In bent-knee postures, keep the knee above or behind the ankle (as in Warrior II, at right).
- In standing postures, stack joints (hips in line with knees and ankles), toes point in same direction as knee
- Avoid hyperextension by micro-bending hyper-mobile joints in all standing poses

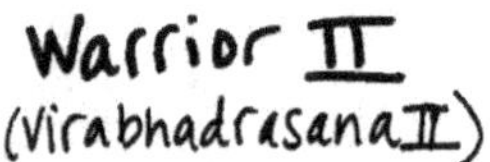

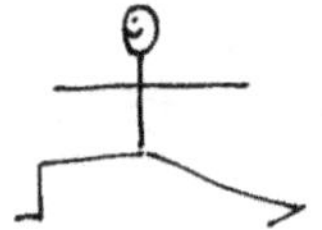

NECK

- Originate twists in the thoracic spine (mid to upper back), allowing your neck and head to be the very last part of your spine to rotate.
- Inversions: use proper support and guidance from a qualified teacher so that weight is never on the neck!

BACK

- In forward bends, fold from the groins/hips, rather than rounding the back.
- A neutral spine has four natural curves (cervical, thoracic, lumbar, sacral). Seek to maintain these curves in virtually every pose.

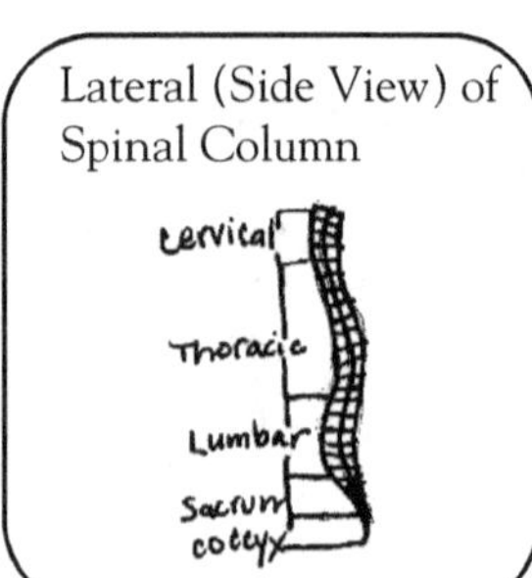

Lateral (Side View) of Spinal Column

FIND CONTENTMENT

In my experience, figuring out how to enjoy each pose is the best strategy to moderate your practice for your own level of flexibility, stamina, and strength. How is this done? Follow these two simple suggestions to bring comfort and ease to your practice:

1. Let your breath be your guide

You should be able to breathe comfortably when practicing yoga. Avoid holding your breath, which sometimes results from too much effort or gripping in the muscles. Instead, go to your edge in a pose and then ease off of it so you can hold the pose comfortably for three breaths or more. Adjusting how deeply you move into a pose will help you find that sweet spot where your body is doing the intended work in the pose without constricting the breath.

2. Use Modifications

Sometimes, during yoga practice, we move our body in ways that are unfamiliar. If we experience sensations that become too strong or painful, our body is telling us that something is not quite right. Use props or other variations, as instructed by a qualified teacher, to experience the pose in a way that creates comfort and ease. Speak up in class if you need help or are uncomfortable in a pose. You'll be glad you did! I know you might feel awkward interjecting, but it is totally appropriate. The only way a teacher will know you need help is if you say something. As the old saying goes, if you have a question, chances are, the other students in the room do too.

YOGA HACK

DIANA'S GUIDELINES FOR SUCCESSFUL YOGA PRACTICE:

- Practice on an empty stomach
- Hydrate early and often
- Every Day, Any Amount
- Observe safe joint alignment
- Find contentment in each pose

A WORD ABOUT THE BREATH

Don't get too hung up on what the breath is doing when you're just beginning your practice. You will first need to learn where your body is and what it's feeling before you can connect your breath with movements. I have some students who struggle to relax into the poses because they are not following the breathing prompts or they are distracted by them. Please allow the breath work to sit on the sidelines and wait for you to get more comfortable with the poses before you pick it up. If you're not confused by it, then by all means, work with it. As you become more experienced, the breathing will become an important part of the practice, but for now, I recommend focusing on the poses.

STICK-TO-ITIVENESS

This guideline is not as formal as some of the others. It's more personal and relates directly to the guidance in this book. I understand starting something new can be hard, and life can easily get in the way. I spoke earlier about keeping your eye on whatever is motivating you to practice, and this section is just a reminder that, **in order to achieve your goal, it will require a bit of "stick-to-itiveness."**

You may think I'm kidding, but I'm not! When you are working on forming a new habit, it is easy to get thrown off course. You're in that sweet spot right between feeling brave for accomplishing something outside of your comfort zone and that space where you own it—where you know it's good for you and you are driven by more than your original purpose to do it. Any little thing can change your trajectory—a family member gets sick, you have important errands to run, your neighbor needs you, your work is getting in the way, etc. And before you know it, you've missed a month of classes. Don't let this be you! Acknowledge that it will take some dedication on your part to guard space in your life to commit to the practice. You will achieve the results you want, but it doesn't happen overnight and it won't happen if you only go to one class, or once a month.

My recommendation as you build a yoga practice into your life is to take it slow, and most importantly, be steady. **The cumulative effects of yoga are amazing, such that the person who practices a little bit every day can get as much or more out of it as the person that practices for one hour twice a week.** Key Point! Keep this in mind as you carve out time and space for the practice. Regularity in smaller batches allows you to make more progress than large chunks of time on an irregular basis. Forming a new habit takes time and effort, and the results won't be instantaneous. Be patient and remain dedicated. You will see the fruits of your labor soon enough.

KEY POINT!

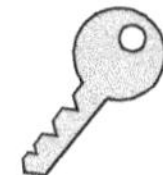 Practicing one yoga pose every day can be as good as or better than practicing for one hour a week.

I know you have it in you to do this. Congratulate yourself for doing things that feel challenging to you, because it prepares you for dealing with all forms of discomfort in your everyday life. Now go ahead and give yourself a pat on the back—you deserve it.

PART 4

MOVING FORWARD

As your stick-to-it-iveness kicks in, the evolution of your practice will naturally move from experimentation to an adoption phase and into an established practice. You might find that you now have a regular practice and a teacher or two you really like. So what's next? What does moving forward look like?

As your practice continues, you might find yourself wanting to practice some on your own. You will memorize the poses such that when you are on vacation or when you first wake up, you will be drawn to do a few poses and realize that you can lead your own short practice at home. Chapter 9 will introduce you to this idea of a personal practice, what it is and how to go about it, right down to the stick figures. I will give you the tools you need to try it out and maybe even integrate yoga into your daily routines. You'll hear my story of how I came to practice at home and ultimately how it shaped my practice going forward.

The final chapter provides some thoughts on deepening your practice. I recommend lots of reflection and further study to accomplish this. One of the added benefits of the practice is the opportunity to get quiet, listen to your body, pay attention to your thoughts and tap in to your own intuition about what your body needs, what you like about the practice, and what you don't like. I'm not here to tell you it is all sunshine and rainbows for every person. You must find what works for you, and there's no better way to know what works than to evaluate your experience and ask more questions.

While we're getting to the end of this book, consider these two final chapters the beginning of the next phase. They are definitely not required reading. Maybe this section should even be the beginning of my next book; *Ready for*

More Yoga. Likewise, I would invite you to skip these chapters and go about enjoying your practice if they do not interest you at the moment. You might find there's a time when your curiosity brings you back to them. They'll be here when you're ready!

Chapter 9
Developing a Personal Practice

As you start your yoga journey, you will be more and more drawn to the practice. For me, it felt almost addictive. Although that's strong language, I did notice, when I first started practicing, that the wonderful feeling I got after practice is what would drive me to practice again. Before long, I would find myself doing a few of the poses first thing in the morning or before my other workouts. The same may likely be true for you. So how do you bridge that gap between practicing weekly with a teacher to doing some on your own? This chapter will guide you through it.

WHAT IS A PERSONAL PRACTICE?

The idea of a personal practice is very simple. Any time you practice any amount of yoga on your own, we call it a "Personal Practice" or sometimes a "Home Practice". This does NOT have to be a big production. In fact, I would argue that you're likely to stick with it and perhaps see greater results if it isn't a big production. You don't need any props, you don't need a quiet space, you don't need an hour, and you don't need yoga pants. All you need is yourself and as little as ten seconds.

Ten seconds. Seriously.

WHY A PERSONAL PRACTICE?

Doing *ANY* amount of yoga every day will bring you closer to your goal more quickly than if you only attend class once or twice a week. A short home practice is another way for you to get some experience in the comfort of your own home without too much effort. And luckily for you, I have the simplest strategy that you can start following immediately. And if you're super excited to drop this book and get started, you can skip forward a few pages to Cat/Cow Pose ("Bidalasana") and have at it. Otherwise, for now, just plant the seed that any amount of yoga every day will propel you forward faster than without it. **Your mantra is "Every Day, Any Amount"**. No matter your goal or interest level, I promise you that "Every Day, Any Amount" will serve you.

KEY POINT!

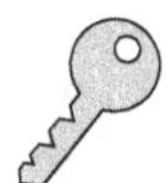 Any amount of yoga every day will set you on a path towards achieving the results you want more quickly.

Have you ever injured yourself and done physical therapy? How often did you see the therapist? And did they expect you to do any of the exercises on your own?

In my experience, physical therapists would like to see patients twice, if not three times a week, and they also expect their patients to do certain exercises at home. They try to make the routines relatively short so this can be accomplished.

Here is one example. When my husband was writing his dissertation, he suffered from incredible carpal tunnel. He found that doing a series of four exercises (30 seconds each) throughout the day (four to six times a day) helped to treat it, as well as prevent further discomfort. Take it from the exercise physiologists—short practices, with frequent repetition, make progress.

MY STORY

I want to share a personal story about how I came to practicing at home on my own, long before being trained as a yoga teacher. My very first yoga teacher, Sean, might be one of the best teachers I've ever had. At the time, I did not know this, of course, as I had not experienced other teachers to be able to compare. And it wasn't until I went through teacher training that I truly realized how wonderful he was. My mother had signed up for a class with him at our local community center. After her first session, she encouraged me to sign up with her. So, at 15, I signed up for my first yoga class. I'll never forget it. I was nervous, for sure. And I do remember it being very challenging.

Sean was trained in the Ashtanga practice, so it was a very athletic experience. My most vivid memory is being in downward-facing dog and my shoulders hurting a lot (I was taking most of the weight in my arms). He gave us a lot of information that we could choose to read in between classes and offered important suggestions like drinking lots of water (he would bring a gallon jug of water with him each time, no lie). I still have his handouts with stick figure drawings of the different poses and he was the inspiration for me to provide my own for students (as you've seen throughout this book).

Once Sean moved to Seattle, my mom and I were a bit lost as far as how to continue with the practice. We didn't have a yoga studio in town, so my mother bought a yoga video with Ali McGraw. We did yoga with that video probably three times a week, to the point where I had it memorized.

Fast forward four years. I was in college, studying abroad in the south of France. It was the most idyllic year, but in many ways very disorienting. At the time, there was no such thing as a student union or athletic facility at the government-run French university in Aix-en-Provence. At the University of Michigan, we had the well-equipped Central Campus Recreation Building (CCRB) where I took hip hop dance and yoga classes. I was used to running and biking and being very physically active. In France, I had to get very creative about exercise. Thankfully, I had Sean's drawings and enough experience with the video that I could practice yoga on my own in my room. Saved!

You might be surprised how often this comes in handy. When traveling or waking up early, get in 15 minutes of practice before starting your day. The longer you practice, the more you'll find an interest in practicing some at home.

WHAT POSES TO PRACTICE

When putting together a home practice, there are essentially two paths: (1) you will either follow a sequence designed by someone else, or (2) you will build your own. I recommend beginning with the former until you gain enough experience to avoid feeling overwhelmed by building your own.

Using stick figure guides was the best way for me to start practicing outside of class. In the next section, I've provided two simple practices to get you going, with stick figure drawings of my own: Cat/Cow Pose and Sun Salutations.

YOGA HACK

More sequences can be found on my website at www.dianashea.com/readyforyoga. Have any questions about them? Email me! info@dianashea.com

---

As you approach these practices, revisit the guidelines of safe alignment for injury prevention in Chapter 8. I must put out a disclaimer that if you try one of these sequences on your own, you are practicing at your own risk. Seeking the help of a qualified teacher to make sure you understand the sequence as I have described it is the best way to ensure your safety.

Lastly, remember that any given practice should ideally be a well-rounded practice (See Chapter 5: Elements of a Well-Rounded Practice for explanation). However, in the spirit of "any amount, every day", please do not let the guidance of "well-rounded" stop you from practicing!

Cat/Cow Pose ("Bidalasana")

In Cat/Cow Pose, you start on hands and knees with your wrists below your shoulders and your knees directly below your hips. We sometimes call this starting position "Table Top Pose". This pose creates length in the spine and can help to prevent, as well as relieve, back pain. It's a very good morning opener pose. We do this by connecting breath with movement as we articulate the flexion and extension of the spine.

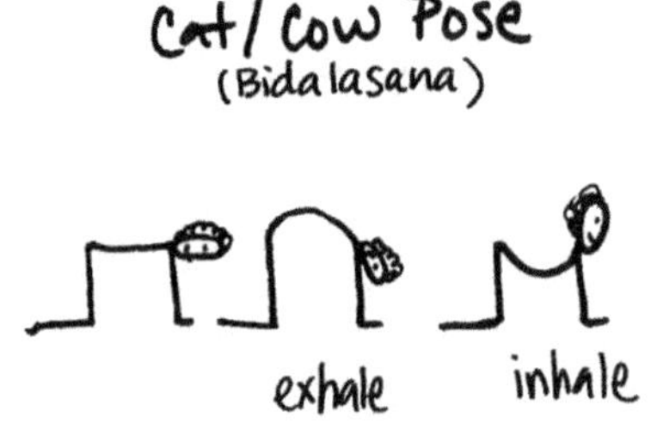

As you exhale, you dome the spine up towards the ceiling like an angry Halloween cat, allowing your head and tailbone to fall towards the mat. On the inhalation, you reverse the motion, allowing the belly to fall towards the mat and look up while the sit bones also go up.

If it is painful for your wrists to be in that much flexion, try elevating your palms by placing them on the rolled front edge of your mat or blanket. Elevate the palms only, leaving the fingers on the mat/floor. If your knees are sensitive in this position, give yourself extra padding by laying a blanket down on the floor or across your mat.

Begin your home practice by doing this one pose. That's it! I'd love it if you did it every day, but if that feels overwhelming, then simply do that pose when you think of practicing some yoga at home. And voila, you have a Home Practice! That's the first step.

Sun Salutation ("Surya Namasakar")

The Sun Salutation is a great sequence to warm up the body for a longer practice or other activities, yet it can also be a stand-alone practice. It is very common for this sequence to be used in a yoga class, so it is worth getting acquainted with it.

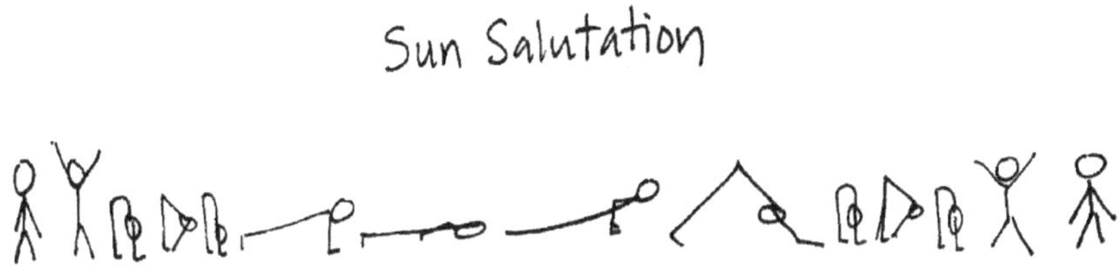

PRIVATE INSTRUCTION

Another way to begin a personal practice is to work with a private teacher. Studying privately with someone, you will be able to customize a sequence to best meet your needs or goals. Working with a teacher to create a plan for your home practice is particularly helpful if you have a specific goal for your practice and would like to see progressive results.

Another reason to work with a professional is for your own accountability. Do you need an appointment (and a payment) in order to create the time and space in your life to do this? Even if it is any amount, every day, some of us need ways to hold ourselves accountable, and working with a private teacher is a very good way to get there.

To find someone to work with, you might follow the same suggestions as outlined in Chapter 6 for finding local classes. Getting feedback from former and current students, as well as interviewing the instructor, is a good idea for setting expectations in an informed way. If you are looking to build your personal practice, be sure to ask for sequences you can practice on your own.

YOGA HACK

Interview questions for private instruction:
• What is your approach to private lessons?
How do you structure the lessons?
• How do you measure growth or progress in the student?
• Tell them your motivation for practice
(check your notebook where you wrote it down)
and the benefits you hope to get out of it.
With that in mind, ask how they would begin.

EVERY DAY, ANY AMOUNT

If I make one thing clear in this chapter, I hope that it is to emphasize that practicing "Every Day, Any Amount" should be your mantra. You will see greater benefit when you practice every day, even if it is for ten seconds or less. Keeping your momentum moving towards the practice and making measurable progress towards functional goals is one reason, and perhaps the primary reason, to practice on a regular (i.e., daily) basis.

But that's not the only reason. **Any teacher will tell you that if you want to learn a new skill, you must practice.** Yoga is no exception. When we first approach yoga, it is messy. You are putting your body into unfamiliar positions and dealing with the discomforts of your own vulnerability as you try something new. It takes a lot of effort and the poses may feel hard, with lots of muscular work. This can distract you from paying attention to the alignment of the pose or understanding the direction of the posture. Taking the time to study some of the postures you learn in class will help you integrate what you're learning. Bringing your awareness to the poses outside the class environment will augment your overall experience. Practice and repetition lead to integration.

KEY POINT!

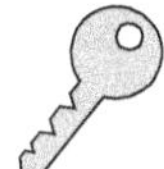

If you want to learn a new skill,
you must practice!

I can vividly remember being in downward-facing dog in that first series class I took with my mom and feeling the weight of my body in my shoulders and wrists. I couldn't believe how long we were holding the pose! I was caught in my own suffering and shut out the experience of the pose itself just to get through it. Practicing the pose at home, I could go in and out of downward-facing dog and play with the pose in a way that was not wrapped up in the stress of keeping up with the class or not knowing what I was doing. I could shift my weight forward and back, and the more I did it, the less effort it required. A self-directed practice creates a different experience.

PERSONAL PRACTICE CHALLENGE

Some say it takes 30 days to create a new habit, so I challenge you to practice "Every Day, Any Amount" for 30 days. Begin today with Cat/Cow pose. Take a selfie and post with #ReadyForYoga30daychallenge. We will all cheer you on!

Chapter 10
Deepening Your Practice

In the study of yoga, there is no beginning and no end. Wherever you start on the path is where you are meant to be. The process of understanding the yoga philosophy and integrating it into your life is an unfolding. As one idea becomes clear, a new question forms. The experience is a series of cycles that lead you down one path of greater depth in a topic, which often circles back to where you began to clarify the starting point. Trust the process and welcome the new experiences and wisdom as you meet them.

For many of us, the process of seeking requires that which we seek. In this case, **finding a way to be comfortable with the unknowing and gradual unfolding is key to staying on the path forward.** That all sounds great, but how do you get there? As with any new experience, a bit of self-reflection, conversation, and exploring further resources will aid you in better understanding what it means for you. Trust the process. Wherever it leads you is where you are supposed to be.

SELF-REFLECTION

Asking ourselves a series of questions to aid in the evaluation of our own experiences is a time-honored technique of conscious living. Writing down the answers to these questions in the form of a journal or discussing them with friends will give you great personal insight. Here are a few prompts to get you started.

REFLECTION QUESTIONS: Answer the questions below to gain insight into how you're doing with your new practice.

Questions for you

1. What is working well for you?
2. What do you like about the practice?
3. What do you not like about the practice?
4. What don't you understand?
5. What would make it better for you?
6. How close are you to achieving your vision for your practice?
7. What adjustments do you need to make to your practice in order to get closer to your vision?
8. Do you have any new beliefs about yoga now that you have some experience/gotten this far in the book?

CONVERSATIONS WITH OTHER STUDENTS

You might remember back in Chapter 6 when I suggested you speak with friends about their experiences in order to find a class. This would be a good time to circle back to those friends and have that conversation again, now that you've taken some classes yourself. Your perspective has shifted and you probably have new questions to ask.

Questions for your friends

1. What style of yoga do you practice? Have you tried any others? How are they different? What do you like and not like about each?
2. How often do you practice?
3. Do you ever practice on your own at home?

CONVERSATIONS WITH YOUR TEACHER

Your yoga teacher is also someone who may now be accessible to you to help clarify some key questions or to help you understand where you are on your path. As a new student, I remember being interested in my teachers and what their experiences were leading up to becoming a teacher. I remember not knowing what to even ask about in order to deepen my own practice. Here are a few prompts to aid you in that conversation, should you choose to approach your teacher.

Questions for your teacher

1. I have really enjoyed this class, where can I learn more about the style?

2. I am interested in deepening my practice, are there any outside resources you would suggest for me? Books, videos, or online? Are there any workshops you would recommend at this point in my practice?

3. The main reason I am practicing yoga is to _______________. What do you think is the best way for me to achieve that? Am I on the right path?

OTHER RESOURCES

When you are ready to learn more, or go deeper into your practice, turning towards books, videos, online content, and workshops is an excellent way to expand your knowledge. Asking your teacher for suggestions will be the best way to find something that speaks directly to your practice and your level of interest. Having in-person experiences first makes a transition to practicing on your own, either with the aid of a book, video, or other resources, safer and easier.

Books

For my students, I recommend *Yoga The Iyengar Way* by Silva, Mira, and Shyam Mehta. This is a large paperback book which has a photo for each pose, along with extremely detailed descriptions. It is a very helpful tool for both new and experienced students. I use it as a reference when studying a certain pose or putting together a sequenced class. It was also one of the textbooks for my teacher training program.

I know other teachers who recommend *The Yoga Bible* by Christina Brown. Similar to the Iyengar book, this one has pictures with detailed descriptions, with more of an emphasis on putting the pieces together and structuring a home practice. It also includes an overview of yoga, much like I've provided in this book.

Online Content

Doing a simple Google search on any yoga topic of interest will bring up a slew of resources, no doubt. It's very hard to determine the quality of a website when you find it this way. Instead, there is another website I would recommend as a good starting point of its own: The Yoga Journal website (http://www.yogajournal.com/). The Yoga Journal is a monthly publication that also has free online content. You can search on that site and find their back articles on a related topic. From there, you might find other reliable references on the topic.

There are some providers of streaming on-demand yoga classes. I would suggest speaking with your teacher about which ones might work well for you.

Series Classes

Signing up for a progressive series class is a great way to expand your practice because of the consistency it provides. A series class is comprised of a set number of classes that you commit to in advance. Participating in a progressive series class gives the teacher the ability to build the lessons from one class to the next and also gives the student an opportunity to commit to the practice by paying in advance for the series.

Workshops

Classes offered in a workshop format are typically longer and focused on a certain topic. Finding a workshop focused on a topic of interest is a wonderful way to gain deeper insight. Workshops can be a few hours, an entire weekend, or sometimes several days. They can be offered in far-off retreat locations (Costa Rica, Mexico, Bali, and India are common ones) or at your local studio. To find an opportunity like this, ask your teacher if they know of any upcoming workshops or retreats they would recommend. You would also find detailed offerings in yoga-specific publications, like *Yoga Chicago*.

Find a new teacher

One easy way to expand your practice is to experience new teachers. This is the simplest method to gain a new perspective. Going to a different class than you are used to will give you a new way to experience the practice. Students that see a sub on the schedule will sometimes avoid coming for fear of the unknown. The teacher is the class and the class is the teacher, and once you get comfortable with one, it is hard to replace them. As humans, we don't like change, but change is how we grow and expand, so it is necessary.

INTEGRATION

Taking the time to reflect on what you're learning, discussing your experience with your community and teacher, and seeking out more information to answer your questions will put you well on your way to integrating yoga into your everyday life. You've learned about where yoga came from, what it can do for you, and how to navigate finding a class. You've experienced some yoga (or plan to soon) and started to create a foundation for your practice.

Looping the practice back into your life will come. One of the unexpected benefits of this practice is that we learn to be kind to ourselves and translate the challenges that we overcome on the mat into our daily life. You will begin to see how the lessons we learn on the mat have real-life applications.

As time goes on and you continue with your practice, remember that your experience is unique to you. Your unfolding and integration of the material into your life is yours and it's serving your best and highest good. Remember that your commitment to yourself and your reasons for practicing are what matters most.

The teacher in me bows to the teacher in you! Namaste.

AFTERWORD

Would you believe my purpose in writing this book is world peace? I could say it is to guide seekers toward the practice, and ultimately toward self-healing, and that, of course, is also true. But when I check in with my gut about why I choose to teach, or why I chose to write this book, it is because our world would be much more fair and kind if there were a successful yoga studio on every corner. I thank Sri Goswami Kriyananda for saying this as part of my teacher training: "Do not worry about competition—the new studio that opens up across from yours—for there ought to be enough demand for yoga to support a studio on every corner." You must try.

At a time when hate seems to be gaining traction in the public discourse in this country, I can only wonder what it would be like if everyone just practiced more yoga. We can all teach kindness, one person at a time. And through this book, hundreds, maybe thousands, or even millions (!) of people may be drawn to the practice. I am hopeful that scaling my impact through this book will be a meaningful contribution.

This book is part of my unfolding—the releasing of all that I have to share with the world that I previously thought was restricted to my yoga classes! I had no idea that I had a book in me until my sister sent me a book called *You Must Write a Book*, followed by another book called *Published*. Through those two books, I realized that I had something to share. And in the writing, I, too, have integrated the knowing in a way that has been unexpected. The path is always unfolding before us.

I remember when I first started my teacher training program, I got a really uncomfortable feeling that there was so much more to know, that my experience with yoga so far was just the tip of the iceberg. This caused frustration. I thought my yoga was one thing and now there was so much more to learn. Thankfully, I was told to trust the process. Today, I am secure in my knowing and recognize that what I need will come to me.

As a teacher, I am also always a student. It's just like parenting. Does the parent teach the child? Or does the child teach the parent? In my experience, both are true. For me, it often feels like my kids are teaching me way more than I ever thought possible. The relationship becomes a beautiful energy exchange without even knowing it. And the process is perfect for both. That's what it is like to teach yoga as well. Find comfort in knowing that, while you may be a new student, your teacher is learning important things from you too.

Ultimately, our yoga practice is a training ground for much more than the poses themselves. Practicing the poses can be a tool to get us to pay attention and take greater responsibility for ourselves, our health and our community. Whether you ask for this or not, it will happen. And that is the beauty! That is how I know that, if I put this out there, not only will you feel great and learn some new skills, you will create ripples of consciousness and kindness that will serve as one big hug for the planet and all of us earthly beings.

GRATITUDE

I extend my deepest gratitude to Goswami Kriyananda, David Lipschutz, Kim Schwartz and The Temple of Kriya Yoga for bestowing upon me the foundation of these teachings. To my students over the years, from Baltimore and Oak Park, you have taught me all that I know.

To my mom, for inviting me to my first yoga class. How did you know it would be good for me? To my sister, Betsy, for having encouraged me to write in the first place. Without your belief in me, it would never have occurred to me to take on this project. To my sister, Katie, for reviewing the earliest draft and giving me her professional opinions along the way. What an honor it has been to have your guidance.

To my husband, Steve, for listening to my daily musings on all that I am seeking and for supporting my desire to live my life by design rather than by default. To my sweet baby girls, Ellie and Sonya, for honoring this endeavor with me and holding my own excitement in your hearts. I share your wonder and delight.

To Steve and Laurie Berggren and the students and staff at The Yoga Centre. Thank you for the opportunity to lead this community of yogis and grow together through fellowship and study.

To all of my family and friends, thank you for showing your excitement over this project that has, hopefully, now inspired you!

APPENDIX A
Movements of the Spine and Limbs

The spine has three types of motion: flexion, extension and rotation. Flexion is forward-folding, extension is back bending, and rotation are twists. For each of these motions, we can cite a variety of examples of standing, seated and supine positions that allow the spine to move in each of these ways.

FLEXION OF THE SPINE

Flexion of the spine is the ability to fold forward. For example, forward flexion of the spine is observed in standing forward fold ("Uttanasana") and seated forward fold ("paschimottanasana").

Seated Forward Fold
(Paschimottanasana)

Standing Forward Fold
(Uttanasana)

EXTENSION OF THE SPINE

Extension of the spine is the opposite of flexion, which we sometimes call back bending. Examples of back bending include the standing balancing pose called Dancer ("Natrajasana"), which allows for a slight, gentle backbend. Another gentle backbend is Locust Pose ("Salabasana").

Dancer Pose
(Natrajasana)

Locust Pose
(Salabhasana)

SPINAL ROTATION

The final movement of the spine is twists, or spinal rotations. A standing spinal twist is Revolved Triangle Pose ("Pavritta Trikonasana"), and a seated twist is a pose dedicated to a Sage called "Maricyasana".

NAME OF A SAGE
(Maricyasana)

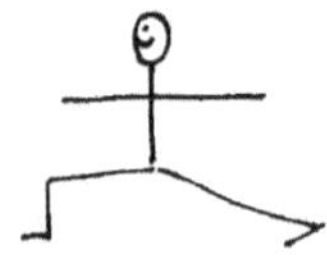

Revolved Triangle Pose
(Pavritta Trikonasana)

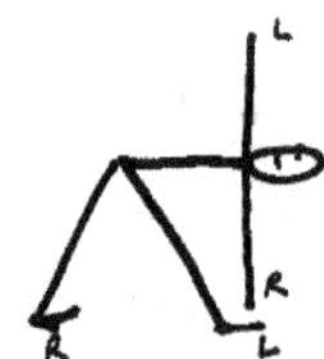

ROTATION OF THE LIMBS

The movements of the limbs in yoga practice include external and internal rotation. External rotation is spiraling the limb away from the midline of the body. If your arms are resting alongside your body, with the palms facing your body, externally rotating the arm will result in the palm facing outward and the thumbs pointing away from the body. Internal rotation is the opposite motion. All the classical postures can be described in these terms. For example, Warrior I ("Virabhadrasana I") is an internally-rotated standing posture with externally-rotated arms. It also has a mild extension of the spine. Using one of the previous examples, Standing Forward Fold ("Uttanasna"), the arms and legs are both internally rotated, and the spine is in flexion.

Warrior II
(Virabhadrasana II)

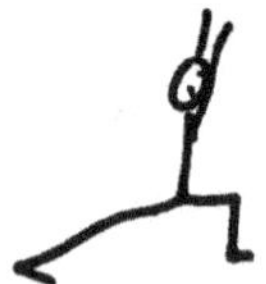

Warrior I
(Virabhadrasana I)

APPENDIX B

Box Breath

One short exercise you can do to bring greater awareness to the breath is called "Box Breath". I have sometimes also heard it referred to as "Square Breath". I offer this as something you can practice on your own in an effort to cultivate greater awareness of your breathing. This is not required—just some extra credit for you. Imagine a square box. Tracing the box with your mind's eye (or a finger, if that's preferred), inhale for four counts as you draw the line up the left side of the box from the bottom to the top. Now as you draw the line from the left of the top to the right, hold the breath for four counts. On the right side of the box, exhale for four counts as you draw the line from the top to the bottom. Lastly, trace the bottom of the box from right to left as you hold for four counts. That is box breathing.

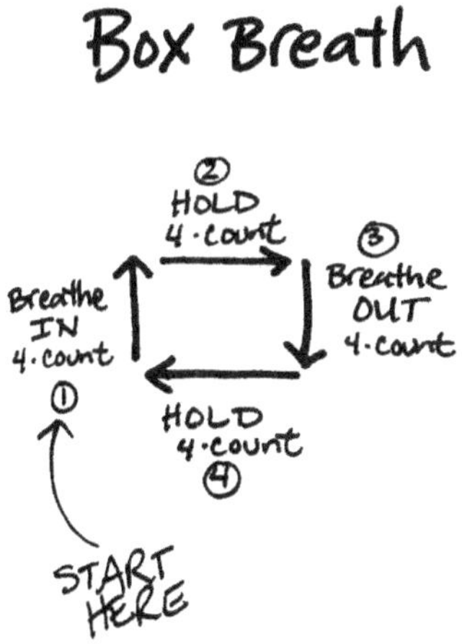

APPENDIX C
Social and Behavioral Guidelines of the Eight Limbs of Yoga

The first two limbs of the eight limbs of yoga are the social and behavioral guidelines. The Sanksrit terms for them are the "Yamas" and the "Niyamas." Each has five guidelines. The tables below describe the guidelines in greater detail. Each of these guidelines can be observed in thought, word and action.

These interpretations of the guidelines come from my own notes and files, however I am not the original author. I cannot take credit for them and regret that I am not able to provide reference details.

The first set of guidelines refers to self-regulating our behaviors involving others. The Sanskrit word for them is "Yama", which means control or restraint. Likewise, the five behaviors defined as "Yamas" are to be restrained: Violence, Lying, Stealing, Sensuality, and Greed. The use of the English translation "Sensuality" often leads to questions. The intention of this guideline is to restrain the senses—to not allow ourselves to be overcome by sensory cravings and to be able to direct our energy in a way that keeps our mind and body in balance or harmony[2].

YAMAS	Behavioral Guidelines to co-exist harmoniously with others	
Sanskrit Word	**Translation**	**Definition**
Ahimsa	Non-Violence	Do not cause harm to yourself or others. Renounce destructive behaviors and thought patterns.
Satya	Non-Lying	Express truthfulness in thought, word and deed. Be authentic.
Asteya	Non-Stealing	Refrain from taking that which has not been earned, as well as that which is not ours.
Brahmacharya	Non-Excess	Become the master of one's creative force. Redirect creative energy by living in
Aparigraha	Non-Greed	Free yourself from that which is not needed.

The second set of guidelines are activities or personal habits that encourage a healthy life in body and mind. They are intended to help find the root of happiness. The Sanskrit word for them is "Niyama", which means without restraint. There are five "Niyamas" or personal disciplines that are to be observed without restraint or limitation: Contentment, Self-Purification, Self-Discipline, Self-Study, and Attunement to Life.

NIYAMA	Personal Disciplines to find the root of happiness	
Sanskrit Word	**Translation**	**Definition**
Santosha	Contentment	State of mind that is at peace with the present moment without being distracted by regrets of the past or hopes for the future.
Saucha	Self-Purification	Clear, focused expression of thought and word. Inner and outer body cleanliness.
Tapas	Self-Discipline	Seeking simplicity and balance through self-discipline.
Svadhayaya	Self-Study	Cultivate self-awareness through continual learning from life's experiences.
Ishvara-pranidhana	Attunement to Life	Evaluate our thoughts, words and deeds in light of how they can reflect our concept of the divine.

APPENDIX D
Creative Childcare Solutions

A creative childcare solution is forming a swap with one or more friends. Do you know anyone else in a similar situation who would like to practice yoga at the same time? Or someone who also needs creative childcare solutions? Link up with them and discuss these possible options, then let your mind run on this as far as other applications for it. Do you need a date night with your spouse and dislike the additional expense of a sitter? I know that's a separate book, but these strategies can have some unrelated benefits. Something to put in the back of your mind.

There are several ways to structure such a swap:

- **Alternate Swap** – form a swap with one other parent or caregiver. One adult goes to yoga, one adult watches the children. The next time, you switch roles.

- **Small Group Swap** – a few parents/caregivers get together, rotating one parent that stays with the kids while the others go practice. Depending on the space available wherever you practice, you could ask if there is room for you to be on-site with the children for logistical ease. Or you could hire your own teacher and bring the class to you! One friend babysits at their house with all the kids while another friend hosts the yoga class.

- **Babysitting Co-Op** – Evenly swap childcare hours with a friend. In this case, the friend might not be interested in going to the same yoga class as you. Perhaps you simply want to set up a direct swap where you share babysitting hours one for one, setting up a weekly schedule. A helpful app for keeping track of this type of swap is iSit.

APPENDIX E
Yoga Alliance Teaching Credentials

The Yoga Alliance is a nonprofit organization that handles credentialing for yoga teachers and schools. There are four levels of teaching designations: RYT 200, E-RYT 200, RYT 500, and E-RYT 500. Please note: **These four categories are not sequential, and in some cases more than one designation is appropriate.** For example, we have one teacher on staff who is both E-RYT 200 and RYT 500. She has the highest level of training (RYT 500) and she has taught at least 1,000 hours.

RYT 200

This is the **primary level of certification**, indicating completion of a registered 200-hour teacher training program. It includes a well-rounded base of yoga practice, teaching methodology, anatomy and physiology, yoga philosophy/ethics/lifestyle, and teaching practicum. These programs tend to provide depth in the techniques of a specific style, rather than a survey of several different ways of teaching. For example, my 200-hour certification was in Hatha Yoga, which did not include much, if anything, about teaching a Vinyasa class. By contrast, the 200-hour teacher training programs at the national chain CorePower Yoga are offered in Power Yoga, Hot Yoga, or Hot Power Fusion.

E-RYT 200

The "E" stands for Experienced. These teachers have completed the RYT 200 level of training and have lots of teaching hours under their belt. More specifically, this designation requires a minimum of two years of teaching experience after completion of the teacher training program and 1,000 teaching hours. Notice that 1,000 teaching hours is no small thing. If a teacher teaches twice a week for 1.5 hours, it would take six years to reach this designation. What this points out is that this level of experience is reserved for those who have set themselves apart with teaching hours.

RYT 500

RYT 500 is the next level of training up from RYT 200. **The "500" indicates that the teacher has completed 500 hours of teacher training instruction in a well-rounded accredited program, regardless of teaching experience.** Likewise, this is the highest level of training, but that doesn't necessarily translate when comparing against teachers with lesser training, but more experience. Is the elementary school teacher with 30 years of experience "better" than the teacher with no teaching experience and a master's degree in education? I don't know, it's hard to say with so little information, but I would tend to believe the experienced teacher would have better results.

E-RYT 500

Again, "E" stands for Experienced. This is the highest yoga teaching designation, including 500 hours of yoga teacher training, four years minimum teaching experience and 2,000 teaching hours. In this case, the teacher is able to dedicate more time to their craft. If they teach four classes per week (each lasting 1.5 hours), it would take them six years after finishing the RYT 500 training in order to achieve E-RYT 500 status. I want to emphasize that these experienced credentials show who is head and shoulders above the rest with the same level of training. **Achieving E-RYT 500 status means this person has made a significant commitment to their teaching.**

END NOTES

[1] YJ Editors (January 13, 2016) 2016 Yoga in America Study. *The Yoga Journal. Retrieved from* https://www.yogajournal.com/page/yogainamericastudy

[2] Amin DJ, Goodman M. The effects of selected asanas in Iyengar yoga on flexibility: pilot study. J Bodyw Mov Ther. 2014 Jul;18(3):399-404. doi:10.1016/j.jbmt.2013.11.008. Epub 2013 Nov 8. PubMed: 25042310.

[3] Ellen Petrick's LinkedIn Profile. Retrieved from https://www.linkedin.com /in/ellen-petrick-9349499/

[5] Innes KE, Bourguignon C, Taylor AG. Risk indices associated with the insulin resistance syndrome, cardiovascular disease, and possible protection with yoga: a systematic review. J Am Board Fam Pract. 2005 Nov-Dec;18(6):491-519. Review. PubMed 16322413.

[6] Cohen DL, Bloedon LT, Rothman RL, Farrar JT, Galantino ML, Volger S, Mayor C, Szapary PO, Townsend RR. Iyengar Yoga versus Enhanced Usual Care on Blood Pressure in Patients with Prehypertension to Stage I Hypertension: A Randomized Controlled Trial. Evid Based Complement Alternat Med. 2011;2011:546428. doi: 10.1093/ecam/nep130. Epub 2011 Feb 14. PubMed 19734256; PubMed Central PMC3145370

[7] Zettergren KK, Lubeski JM, Viverito JM. Effects of a yoga program on postural control, mobility, and gait speed in community-living older adults: a pilot study. J Geriatr Phys Ther. 2011 Apr-Jun;34(2):88-94. doi: 10.1519/JPT.0b013e31820aab53. PubMed 21937898.

The study's conclusion states: "The yoga program designed for this study included the activities of standing, sitting, and lying on the floor. Therefore, subjects perform activities during yoga that can improve postural control, mobility, and gait speed."

[8] Polsgrove MJ, Eggleston BM, Lockyer RJ. Impact of 10-weeks of yoga practice on flexibility and balance of college athletes. Int J Yoga. 2016 Jan-Jun;9(1):27-34. doi: 10.4103/0973-6131.171710. PubMed 26865768; PubMed Central PMC4728955.

Note: Using college male athletes, this study looked at athletes that practiced yoga 2x/week over 10 weeks, and those that did no yoga in addition to their other fitness activities. The yoga group showed significant increase in flexibility and balance as measured by sit and reach, shoulder flexibility, stork stand and changes in joint angles when practicing three distinct yoga poses (down dog, chair pose, right foot lunge).

[9] Streeter CC, Whitfield TH, Owen L, Rein T, Karri SK, Yakhkind A, Perlmutter R, Prescot A, Renshaw PF, Ciraulo DA, Jensen JE. Effects of yoga versus walking on mood, anxiety, and brain GABA levels: a randomized controlled MRS study. J Altern Complement Med. 2010 Nov;16(11):1145-52. doi: 10.1089/acm.2010.0007. Epub 2010 Aug 19. PubMed 20722471; PubMed Central PMC3111147.

[10] Streeter CC, Gerbarg PL, Whitfield TH, et al. Treatment of Major Depressive Disorder with Iyengar Yoga and Coherent Breathing: A Randomized Controlled Dosing Study. Journal of Alternative and Complementary Medicine. 2017;23(3):201-207. doi:10.1089/acm.2016.0140.

Note: Depressive symptoms were significantly decreased in both the high-dose yoga group (3 90-minute weekly Iyengar yoga sessions plus homework) and the low-dose yoga group (2 90-minute weekly Iyengar yoga sessions plus homework)

[11] 1: Blumenthal JA, Emery CF, Madden DJ, George LK, Coleman RE, Riddle MW, McKee DC, Reasoner J, Williams RS. Cardiovascular and behavioral effects of aerobic exercise training in healthy older men and women. J Gerontol. 1989 Sep;44(5):M147-57. PubMed 2768768.

The study concluded, "Although few significant psychological changes could be attributed to aerobic exercise training, participants in the two active treatment groups perceived themselves as improving on a number of psychological and behavioral dimensions."

[12] 1: Ross A, Thomas S. The health benefits of yoga and exercise: a review of comparison studies. J Altern Complement Med. 2010 Jan;16(1):3-12. doi: 10.1089/acm.2009.0044. Review. PubMed 20105062.

[13] Feuerstein, Georg The Yoga Tradition Prescott, AZ : Hohm Press, 1998

[14] The Eight Limbs of Yoga in English and their original Sanskrit names:

1. THE DONT'S ("YAMA")
2. THE DO'S ("NIYAMA")
3. THE POSES ("ASANA")
4. BREATH CONTROL ("PRANAYAMA")
5. SENSE WITHDRAWAL ("PRATYAHARA")
6. CONCENTRATION ("DHARANA")
7. MEDITATION ("DHYANA")
8. ENLIGHTENMENT ("SAMADHI")]

[15] In some cases, you will hear this referred to as 'Enlightenment'.

[16] *Anusara School of Hatha Yoga* Retrieved from https://www.anusarayoga.com/philosophy/

[17] *Anusara School of Hatha Yoga* Retrieved from https://www.anusarayoga.com/teacher-support/key-elements-of-an-anusara-yoga-class/

[18] Baumeister, Roy F.; Finkenauer, Catrin; Vohs, Kathleen D. (2001). "Bad is stronger than good" (PDF). Review of General Psychology. 5 (4): 323–370. doi:10.1037/1089-2680.5.4.323. Retrieved 2014-11-19.

Pratto, Felicia; Oliver, John P. (1991). "Automatic vigilance: The attention-grabbing power of negative social information". Journal of Personality and Social Psychology. 61 (3): 380–391. 1941510. doi:10.1037/0022-3514.61.3.380. Retrieved 2014-11-20.

Bergeisen, M (September 22, 2010). The Neuroscience of Happiness. Greater Good Magazine. Retrieved from https://greatergood.berkeley.edu/article/item/the_neuroscience_of_happiness

[19] Sovik, R (Feb 11, 2014). Brahmacharya: The Middle Path of Restraint. Yoga International. Retrieved from https://yogainternational.com/article/view/brahmacharya-the-middle-path-of-restraint. This is a particularly accessible article on the concept of Brahmacharya and contemporary application of it.